CHOLESCINTIGRAPHY

DEVELOPMENTS IN NUCLEAR MEDICINE

VOLUME 1

Cholescintigraphy

edited by

P.H. COX
Rotterdamsch Radio-Therapeutisch Instituut
Department of Nuclear Medicine
Rotterdam

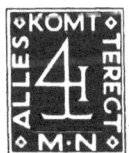

1981

MARTINUS NIJHOFF PUBLISHERS
THE HAGUE / BOSTON / LONDON

Distributors

for the United States and Canada
Kluwer Boston, Inc.
190 Old Derby Street
Hingham, MA 02043
USA

for all other countries
Kluwer Academic Publishers Group
Distribution Center
P.O. Box 322
3300 AH Dordrecht
The Netherlands

ISBN-13:978-94-009-8327-4   e-ISBN-13:978-94-009-8325-0
DOI: 10.1007/978-94-009-8325-0

Copyright © 1981 by Martinus Nijhoff Publishers, The Hague.
Softcover reprint of the hardcover 1st edition 1981

CONTENTS

FOREWORD

This book is timely and fills a void in the area of cholescintigraphy in Nuclear Medicine. It is true that many articles and papers from symposia on this subject are available but they are all scattered through a volumnous literature. Dr Cox and his colleagues have brought together in an orderly fashion the current available material on hepatobiliary scintigraphy in an excellent volume suitable for both the clinician as well as the clinical scientist.

This volume begins with a detailed discussion of anatomy and physiological functions of the liver and biliary tract followed by a section on scintigraphic functional imaging of the liver. A description of the chemistry and pharmaceutical considerations of Tc^{99m} labeled hepatobiliary agents, especially those of Ida-derivatives is included. Next the text follows the usual pattern of discussion on the pharmacodynamics of radiopharmaceuticals, followed by a description of various clinical disease patterns of the liver and the use of cholescintigraphy in evaluating these diseases. The last sections deal with computer applications in quantitation of liver function followed by a discussion of the clinical role for Tc^{99m} labeled hepatobiliary agents in comparison to ultrasonography, CT, radiography and in vitro laboratory tests.

One notable feature of this book is its discussion on the evaluation of new agents in normal experimental animals and in animals with induced liver disease, correlating this data to define the best radiopharmaceutical and then evaluating the same in patients. This type of methodological treatment of the subject matter is commendable.

This volume also reflects the change in the conduct of nuclear imaging from an organ imaging concept to dynamic functional imaging. Hepatobiliary studies using Tc^{99m} labeled radiopharmaceuticals have really opened up a new area of imaging and quantitation of hepatocyte function. Newer agents may fulfill this latter objective more effectively.

To help clinicians from various other disciplines, Nuclear Medicine physicians must find out where scintigraphic methods can eliminate diagnostic uncertainties better than other approaches. They must also know the various drawbacks and pitfalls associated with every Nuclear Medicine procedure. Books like this one can help Nuclear Medicine clinicians in that respect. Certainly this text discusses the fundamentals, clinical applications and more importantly the limitations of cholescintigraphy in Nuclear Medicine. Dr Cox and his colleagues have clearly provided an excellent perspective on this subject.

Gopal Subramanian, Ph.D.
Professor of Radiology
Upstate Medical Center
Syracuse, New York U.S.A.

ACKNOWLEDGEMENTS

The willing collaboration of my fellow contributors made the realization
of this book possible in a short period of time to ensure that it is as up to
date as possible.

A great many people, many unknown to me, have contributed by preparing
illustrations. In this respect I would like to acknowledge the contributions
of Mr. L. Ries, Mr. H. Vuik and Ir. H. Delhez.
Further Mrs. E.L.A. Vonk-Neele and Mrs. M. Westerhout-Kersten for their help
in verifying literature sources. Mrs. M.J.M.C. Busker prepared the manuscript
in its final form, to her a special word of thanks. Finally the collaboration
of Martinus Nijhoff B.V. is greatfully acknowledged.

P.H. Cox.

Contributors:

- **H.J. BIERSACK**

  Institut für Nuklearmedizin der Universität
  Bonn-Venusberg 1

- **P.H. COX**

  Rotterdamsch Radio- Therapeutisch Instituut
  Rotterdam

- **G. FUEGER**

  Universitätsklinik für Radiologie
  Landeskrankenhaus
  Graz

- **H.G. REICHELT**

  St. Franziskushospital
  Bielefeld

- **H.S.L.M. TJEN**

  Rotterdamsch Radio- Therapeutisch Instituut
  Rotterdam

INTRODUCTION

The importance of the liver has long been recognized. Around 2000 BC the Sumarians reported it as being a collecting centre for blood and therefore the seat of life. This point of view was assimilated into the Assyrian and Babylonian cultures and in Plato's timaeus the liver is described as mirror reflecting the thought of the intelligent spirit which appeared to have a moral function and was influenced by bile and sweetness.

In twentieth century western medicine the liver is still regarded as being the seat of life but for different reasons and much time and energy has been utilized to develop ways and means of evaluating liver function.

The use of scintigraphy to visualize the liver is a well known and trusted technique. This has primarily been centred around the use of radioactive colloidal substances which accumulate in the Kupffer cells. For a variety of technical reasons reagents, such as Iodinated rose bengal and bromsulphophtalein which localize in hepatocytes have been little used.

In recent years, however, the development of Technetium labeled compounds which accumulate in hepatocytes and are rapidly excreted in the bile have represented a potential major breakthrough in the use of non-invasive methods for the investigation of liver disease. Of these reagents the most widely used have been derivatives of iminodiacetic acid (IDA) and in particular Diethylida.

By following the biological distribution of this reagent with time by means of serial scintigrams obtained with a gamma camera and by recording quantitative information in the form of time activity curves or functional images it is possible to obtain macroscopic information concerning liver morphology, to demonstrate biliary obstruction and to evaluate hepatocyte function in one study.

In this volume the scientific basis of cholescintigraphy has been outlined together with the application of this knowledge to the clinical situation. The results have been compared with those obtained using other diagnostic methods to demonstrate its value to the clinician especially in the study of the highly jaundiced patient when other studies may be of little value or even contraindicated.

There is little doubt that cholescintigraphy has not yet reached its full potential. We hope that this volume will stimulate the optimum usage of this technique by providing a comprehensive basis upon which clinicians can form their own opinions.

P.H. Cox.

1. THE LIVER AND BILIARY TRACT. ANATOMICAL AND PHYSIOLOGICAL CONSIDERATIONS

H.S.L.M. TJEN

1.1. The liver

The liver is the largest organ in the body weighing in the adult of 1200-1500 g comprising one fiftieth of the total body weight. It is located in the upper part of the abdomen where it occupies the right hypochondriac and the greater part of the epigastric region. A part of its surface is associated with the diaphragm. The location of the liver is dependent on the position of the body and varies with respiration. The topography is altered in some diseases and can be changed by displacement of the organ due to thoracic processes which may push the liver downwards (1). In contrast to the multilobulated liver of many mammals, the human liver is a compact and continuous mass of parenchyma. There are two anatomically distinct lobes, divided conventionally by the line of insertion of the falciform ligament. The right lobe is larger than the left lobe and has on its posterior-inferior surface two smaller lobes: the caudate and the quadrate lobes. The whole organ is covered by the fibrous capsule of Glisson. In the porta hepatis which is situated on the visceral surface of the right lobe, the branches of the hepatic artery and portal vein enter the liver and the common bile duct leaves the liver. At this point the capsule of Glisson enters into the liver following the blood vessels and biliary ducts.

The liver plays an important role in the intermediate metabolism and storage of carbohydrates, the metabolism of fats and amino-acids and the synthesis of proteins. It serves as a depository for numerous vitamins, enzymes and hormones and a large number of chemical syntheses are carried out. Bile is secreted into the bile ducts, synthetized from bile-salts and bile pigments.

The mammalian liver is made up of polygonal prisms, each representing a defined unit known as a lobule. Hepatic lobules were already discribed by Malpighi (2) in 1666 and Mascagni (3) in 1819. A more definite concept of hepatic lobulation as basic architecture was introduced by Kiernan (4) in 1833 who described the hexagonal lobule centered around the radicles of the hepatic veins. Running through the center of the lobule along its longitudinal axis, is the central vein. At the periphery are situated the branches of the portal vein (intra-lobular vein), the interlobular bile ducts, branches of the hepatic artery and the lymphatics, which form a network about the portal vein and its branches. Many authors however have questioned the existence of the classic hexagonal lobule (5,6,7,8,9). Rappaport described acinar units and demonstrated that a lobule is centered around a terminal portal venule and adjoined at its periphery by one or more hepatic veins (10). Scanning electron microscopy of the liver confirmed this finding (11).

The plates of liver cells are separated from one another by the The lining of the hepatic sinusoids is composed of an irregular alternation of two kinds of cells connected by many intermediate forms. One of these two lining cells are fixed macrophages, the phagocytic stellate cells of Von Kupffer which may contain phagocytosed material (12).

1.2. The blood supply of the liver

The importance of blood flow for hepatic function has long been appreciated and much attention has been given to methods of measurement. Abnormalities of the hepatic circulation cause reduced hepatocyte uptake capacity (13).

The liver circulation is characterized by its dual blood supply. It receives blood from the hepatic artery and the portal vein, which latter transports blood that has already passed through the capillaries of the gastro-intestinal tract and the spleen. The terminal vessels of the hepatic artery enter the portal fissure and follow the branches of the portal vein quite closely. The distribution of the vascular tree is just like the biliary tree within the liver and is strictly segmental. The hepatic arterial and the portal venous streams meet in the lateral portions of the liver lobules, where they enter the sinusoids. This mixed blood proceeds through these wide channels to the center of the lobule and enters the branches of the hepatic veins. After a short course it joins the inferior caval vein (14,15,16,17). By means of the Fick principle reliable estimates of the flow through the liver are possible, also (18,19,20,21,22,23) used infusion of bromsulphalein for the estimation of blood flow. Somewhat better is the estimation of blood flow by means of indocyanine green as described by Caesar (19) but a disadvantage is the instability of this compound in plasma. Radionuclides have also been used to estimate blood flow: ^{131}I-Rose Bengal was used by Winkler (22). In 1962 Ueda (24) used [198]Au for the determination of the ratios of flow through the hepatic arterial and portal vein. Pabst et al (25) found the clearance of radioactive gold to be useful for

measuring liver blood flow. Rees (20) and Mackenzie (23) described the use of
^{133}Xenon for this purpose.

1.3. The liver cell

The liver cells are arranged more or less regularly in columns extending
radially from the central vein to the periphery of the lobule. In adults fine
bile canaliculi run between the hepatic cells and form a condensation of the
membrane of the hepatic cells (7). The structure and function of the hepatocyte
is mostly polarized: materials are absorbed from the blood at the sinusoidal
surfaces and bile constituents are secreted at the surfaces exposed to the bile
canaliculi (26). Damage to the liver cell can therefore impair its function in
two directions each independent of the other. The cytoplasm of the liver cell
presents an extremely variable appearance which reflects to some extent the
functional state of the cell.

The extensive use of electron microscopy correlated to cytochemical and
histiochemical analysis has resulted in a new dimension in the understanding of
liver disease in that disorders of organelles of the cells are being recognized.
The absorptive and secretory surfaces of the liver cells are increased by the
microvilli, projected into the lumen of the bile canaliculi and peri-sinusoidal
tissue space (26,27). The mitochondria are the main and probably exclusive sites
of oxidative phosphorylations (26), glycogeen synthesis also occurs there. In
1918 Cowdry (28) stressed already that mitochondria are much more sensitive
indicators of cell damage than are nuclei. This statement has been confirmed by
others (29,30). The endoplasmatic reticulum is a system of submicroscopic tubuli
and flattened vesicles in the cytoplasma. It is possible to distinguish between a
rough or granular reticulum and a smooth or agranular reticulum. The first is
responsible for the synthesis of albumin and some globulins including fibrino-
gen (31). It has a high content of RNA. The latter has great importance for
glycogenesis as pointed by Porter (32,33). Further it is the site for bilirubin
conjugation and detoxification of many drugs and other foreign compounds (34).
Other intrecellular structures are the lysosomes: pericanalicular dense bodies
adjacent to the bile canaliculi (35). The nucleus containing DNA and the Golgi
apparatus, which is also situated near the canaliculi and plays a role in the
secretion of ingested material (36).

1.4. The biliary system

The biliary system commences with the intercellular bile capillaries and canaliculi which empty into the smallest bile ducts. Ellinger and Hurt (37) first visualized the bile capillaries with fluorescence microscopy. The bile capillaries form an intercommunicating network within the center of the liver cell plates and appear to lie within grooves in them, though they actually constitute a part of them. The network of bile canaliculi drains to the smallest intralobular bile ducts, the cholangioles. In the portal tracts the cholangioles communicate with the smallest interlobular bile ducts. When the ducts become wider due to confluence of the smaller ones and approach the hilus, their epithelium becomes high columnar and mucus producing. The right and left lobar ducts which leave the liver in the porta hepatis become the right and left hepatic ducts and fuse to form the common hepatic ducts with a length of 2-3 cm. After the common duct is joined by the cystic duct on its right side, it forms the common bile duct. The normal internal biliary duct pressure is regulated by the secretory pressure of the liver, the distensibility of the gall-bladder and the resistance of the choledochal and ampullary sphincters (38). Recent studies have shown that there is no peristalsis in the common bile duct, only a milking action of the several sphincter muscles at its distal end (39,40). The physio- logical regulation of the flow bile into the duodenum can be thought of as the result of a balance between two types of pumps and one major resistance (41). The principal resistance to bile is provided by the sphincter of Oddi. Neural and hormonal stimuli can increase the flow of bile by contracting the gall- bladder and relaxing the sphincter of Oddi (42).

1.5. The gall-bladder

The gall-bladder is a pear-shaped, hollow structure, closely attached to the posterior surface of the liver. It consists of a fundus, a body and a neck which progresses into the cystic duct. It shows marked variations in shape and size and is frequently the site of pathological processes which change the size and thickness of the wall. The major functions of the gall-bladder are to concentrate and store bile and to deliver it to the duodenum during meals. When stimulated by cholecystokinine the gall-bladder also delivers the concentrated bile through the cystic duct into the common bile duct and the intestine (43). The mechanism of concentrating bile is an active process in and through the wall of the gall-bladder which absorbs fluid and electrolytes (44,45).

1.6. Bile formation and secretion of organic compounds in bile

Bile is produced in man at the rate of 15 ml per kg body weight in 24 hours (46,47). Total bile flow is largely determined by the flow of the blood through the liver (48). Bile flow varies with the portal blood flow, although sudden interruption of the latter decreases, but does not stop bile flow. In first instance the relationship between blood flow and bile production is controlled by hepatic cell function. The total amount of what is produced is defined by bile secretion in the canaliculi, in the ducti and by the biliary system (49). Bile acids induce bile flow, i.e. they induce fluid movement during their secretion into the biliary canaliculi (50,51,52) and it has been proved that the initial phase of the formation of bile is the active transport of bile-acids from parenchymal cells into the bile canaliculi. The osmotic effect of these substances results in a flow of water and solutes into the bile canaliculi. The total amount of bile that finally reaches the duodenum is further dependent on the entero-hepatic cycle of the bile acids (53,54).

Much of what we know about the secretion of bile originates from observing the livers of animals following the administration of fluorescent dyes (Grafflin (55), Mendeloff (56), Hanzon (57), described the behaviour of the dye sodium-fluorescein:

- within 3-10 seconds after intravenous injection the dye appears in the blood plasma of the hepatic sinusoids, then in the Kupffer cells and after 15-32 seconds traces of the dyes are found within the liver cell. Bile canaliculi contain the dye 26-27 seconds after it reaches the sinusoids. In 30-60 minutes the liver cells are cleared of the dye, although it can be detected in the canaliculi as long as two hours after injection.

In the last years kinetic analysis has been carried out with radioactive tagged substances (58,59). When the excretion of bile is abruptly interrupted by mechanical obstruction of the bile ducts, bile continues to be formed and is absorbed from the liver at first through the lymphatics and later by the blood vessels of the liver (57). Hanzon (57) suggests a leakage from the bile canaliculi into the blood, either between or through the liver cells. Leakage most often develops in injured liver cells of which the permeability has been altered because of the raised pressure in bile ducts. However the toxic action of a high consentration of bile acids may be important. In prolonged biliary obstruction there is an astonishing degree of biliary hyperplasia and liver cell atrophy, perhaps due to chemical irritation, that commences within a few days of obstruction (47).

Organic substances can enter the bile by diffusion, secretion or filtration. Mechanisms by which many substances enter the bile are closely associated

with the mechanism of bile formation (51). Extracellular fluid to cell transfer
may consist of active transport, facilitated by diffusion, pinocytosis or a
combination of these processes. Accumulation within the cell often results from
binding to cell components and it is possible that active transport contributes
to the accumulation (60). The nature of the transfer process is determined by
the kind of organic compound.

1.7. Types of compound present in bile

Two kinds of substances are present in hepatic bile.

1. Those which are found in concentrations that differ slightly from those found
   in plasma; they represent a protein free ultrafiltrate of plasma formed by
   the liver cells. The chief examples are Na^+, K^+, Cl^-, creatinine, glucose and
   cholesterol (47).
2. Others such as bilirubin and p-aminohippurate, are much more strongly
   concentrated in bile than in plasma and reach the bile by an active secretory
   mechanism. In addition bile acids are secreted after their synthesis by liver
   cells.

ad 1

The organic compounds which appear in bile in a concentration similar to or
smaller than in plasma include lipid-insoluble molecules, highly lipid soluble
weak electrolytes and a miscellaneous group or organic ions. Studies of the
hepatic uptake and biliary excretion of lipid-soluble drugs are complicated by
the fact that most of these substances are metabolized by the liver (61). Large,
lipid-insoluble molecules enter the bile via restricted diffusion or filtration
(62). Large insoluble molecules could enter the liver cells either by diffusing
through pores in the cell membrane, or by being taken up by some non-specific
transport process such as pinocytosis (63,64). An alternative pathway for these
substances from extracellular fluid to bile would be through intracellular
spaces (62). When this latter pathway may be open to all substances it is to a
degree dependent on the size of molecules.

ad 2

The compounds which appear in bile in a concentration greatly exceeding that of
plasma, are transfered against a sizeable concentration gradient and have to pass
at least two membranes between plasma and the bile: a substrate must penetrate
a liver cell before it can be secreted into bile. Therefore there is strong
evidence that plasma-to-cell and cell-to-bile transfer takes place by a process
of active transport. Mendeloff (56) showed an accumulation of Rose Bengal in

hepatic parenchymal cells. The cellular accumulation of fluorescein appears to be highly dependent on temperature variations, therefore this characteristic might be accepted as evidence that accumulation results mainly from active transport. Some investigations have shown that secreted compounds as brom-sulphalein and procaine amide ethobromide are bound to components of liver tissue (65,66). It seems clear that cellular accumulation of these substances is is due, at least in part, to binding; but this does not rule out the possible participation of active transport in the overall accumulation in vivo. Levi et al (67) demonstrated that the liver cell contains two plasma protein fractions which they called Y-protein and Z-protein. These proteins play an important role in the selective uptake of organic anions by the liver cell. Solomon (65) and Schanker (68) described a study of the uptake of procaine by rat liver slices. Although this compound is bound to some extent by tissue components, it appears to become concentrated in the slice mainly by a process of active transport.

Bilirubin is an example of an organic anion, actively secreted into bile. An immense body of literature has accumulated since Staedeler (69) coined the name bilirubin in 1864. The first bilirubin determination for clinical use was developed by Ehrlich (70) in 1883 and Hijmans van den Bergh (71) distinguished the direct and indirect bilirubin reaction. In 1953 Cole et al (72) found the bilirubin conjugated with glucuronic-acid connected with the direct bilirubin reaction of Hijmans van den Bergh (71) and the unconjugated bilirubin connected with the indirect reaction of Hijmans van den Bergh. Of the bilirubin produced daily, 80% orginates from haemoglobin in the erythrocytes demolished in the reticulo-endothelial cells. In serum the unconjugated bilirubin is present in the albumin form (73). Less than 1 per cent of the total amount of unconjugated bilirubin is present in the blood in its free form, i.e. not bound to albumin. Under pathological conditions the amount of free bilirubin can increase. The liver cell plays a complex role in the bilirubin metabolism (74). Dissociation of the bilirubin-albumin complex may occur on or along the liver cell membrane (75). Intracellular proteins (67) play a very important role in the selective uptake by the liver cell. In de endoplasmic reticulum the conjugation process of bilirubin takes place by means of the enzyme glucuronyl-transferase; the activated glucuronide is derived from glucose (76). The conjugating capacity of the liver cell is unlimited, but the excretory capacity for conjugated bili-rubin has limits (77). There is no precise knowledge concerning the mechanism by which the liver excretes the bilirubin. The great majority of bilirubin is excreted by the liver in the form of water soluble diglucoronide (78). Secretion of bile acids determines the excretion; also hormones such as secretine play an important role (79).

1.8. Some pathophysiological considerations

Disease of liver and biliary tract. Although the liver has already attracted much attention and has been in the past a subject for detailed study by physicians in most areas of medicine, many problems concerning the liver have not yet been resolved. A worth while historical review concerning the liver and jaundice has been written by Moulin (80). Disorders of the liver and biliary system may occur in hepatic cells, the reticulo-endothelial system and the vascular system or bile ducts. In general disorders of liver and biliary system can be classified as jaundiced or non-jaundiced with or without pain. Each condition may be reflected in one or more typical patterns associated with diagnostic methods as biochemical tests, needle biopsy, radiological and radio-isotopes investigations. However the case history, the clinical picture and the observations made during the physical examination may also play an important role in the differential diagnosis of liver and biliary tract disease.

1.9. Cholestasis

Cholestasis is a visible stagnation of bile pigment in bile canaliculi, hepatocytes and in Kupffer cells (81). It can also be defined as a failure of normal amounts of bile to reach the duodenum (82), or a disturbance of hepato-cytic secretion of bile (83). Cholestasis may be produced by a number of factors. Extrahepatic cholestasis is caused by complete or incomplete obstruc-tion of the extrahepatic biliary passage in an axis from the papilla of Vater to the bifurcation of the main hepatic duct at the hilus of the liver. Obstruction of only one part of the intrahepatic biliary duct system, even if including a main branch of the duct only exceptionally leads to jaundice. Biochemical alterations associated with obstruction are usually found. Clinical and laborat-ory manifestations of cholestasis, without demonstrable obstruction on surgical exploration or cholangiography, is one of the main problems in the differential diagnosis of jaundice. This condition is termed intrahepatic cholestasis. Whatever may be the cause of cholestasis, the hepatocyte changes may be the same. The characteristic picture of severe cholestasis may present in various forms with absence of portal inflammation or with a severe inflammatory reaction (84). Examination by electron microscopy demonstrated alterations not only in the bile canaliculi, but also in hepatocellular organelles throughout the lobule

(85) in all forms of cholestasis. Even electron microscopy does not detect any difference between the lesions produced by mechanical obstruction and the primary form of cholestasis. Desmet (86) suggested therefore that the differential diagnosis is not based on the functional or structural evaluation of the cholestasis, but rather on appreciation of the accompanying features such as inflammation or the type of cell damage, the etiology or the empiric knowledge of the course of development of the condition.

1.10.Mechanism of cholestasis

The initial element in the development of extrahepatic cholestasis is obviously obstruction in the bile ducts. Secondary events within the liver cell are then initiated and a secondary intrahepatic cholestasis is produced which in its turn leads to the same symptoms (83). At its origin in the liver the biliary system is a closed system. Under normal circumstances the conjugated bilirubin excreted by the liver cell into this system, cannot escape and can only be transported to the intestinal tract. When an obstruction in the biliary system exists the permeability of the biliary tree may alter and bilirubin can then pass into the blood (87). The wall of the intercellular capillaries is formed by the liver cells themselves. When damage to the liver parenchyma occurs the integrity of the intrahepatic biliary tree is destroyed and bilirubin excreted in the bile capillaries, can also leak into the blood. In intrahepatic cholestasis the primary cause is generally obscure but again secondary changes follow within the liver cell itself. Up to now the mechanism whereby this occurs has not been established although there have been many hypotheses. Schaffner and Popper (88) described a dysfunction of smooth endoplasmatic reticulum whilst mitochondrial and canalicular membrane injury has been described by Schersten (89) and Ozawa et al (90) reported about the hypothesis that cholestasis may result either from a disturbance of the systems responsible for solute transport into the bile canaliculi ("solute pumps") or from an alteration of canalicular microvilli.

1.11.Pathology

All of changes observed are time dependent. In cholestasis conventional microscopy shows accumulation of bile in liver cells, Kupffer cells and the canaliculi (91). Biliary cirrhosis results from prolonged cholestasis. In extrahepatic cholestasis dilated intrahepatic ducts and a proliferation and dilatation of marginal bile ducts in the edematous portal zone can be observed (92).

In intrahepatic cholestasis multiplied bile ducts are not seen, but liver cell damage is always present.

1.12.Classification of cholestasis (88)

A. Cholestasis produced by demonstrable obstruction of the bile ducts

1. extrahepatic obstruction: (obstacle to bile flow in the common hepatic duct of common bile duct between the papilla of Vater and bifurcation within the liver)

- gall-stones
- tumours
- inflammatory lesions of the bile ducts associated with strictures:
 - post surgical
 - sclerosing cholangitis
- pancreatic disease
- various causes:
 - choledochal cysts
 - amoebic abcesses
 - diverticula of the duodenum
 - parasitic infection
 - haemobilia
 - inspissatio bile syndrome
 - fibrosis of the sphincter of Oddi

2. intrahepatic obstruction: (diffuse or focal obstruction of intrahepatic bile ducts)

- carcinoma of the bifurcation of the common hepatic duct
- infantile obstructive cholangiopathy
- intrahepatic cholangitis
- periductal and periductural fibrosis
- metastatic carcinoma
- polycystic liver disease

B. Cholestasis without demonstrable biliary obstruction (intrahepatic chole-stasis)

1. hepatitis:

- viral hepatitis
- alcoholic hepatitis
- drug hepatitis

2. pure interhepatic cholestasis:

- haemolytic conditions
- cholestasis complicating infections
- alpha-1-antitrypzine defency
- congestive cholestasis
- amyloïdosis
- malignancies including lymphoma
- cholestasis of pregnancy
- idiopathic recurrent intrahepatic cholestasis
- drug induced cholestasis (without hepatitis)
- progressive familial cholestasis in children

REFERENCES

1. Villemin F, Dufour R, Rigaud A: Variations morphologiques en topographiques du foie. Arch. Mal. Appar. dig. 40:63, 1951.

2. Malpighi M, De viscerum structura exercitatio anatomica. London, 1666.

3. Masgagni P, Prodromo della granda Anatomia. Firenze, 1819.

4. Kiernan F, The anatomy and physiology of the liver. Philosoph. Tr. Roy. Soc. London, 123:711, 1833.

5. Mall FP, A study of the structural unit of the liver. Amer. J. Anat. 5:227, 1906.

6. Arey LB, On the presence of so-called portal lobules in the seal's liver. Anat. Rec. 51:315, 1932.

7. Elias H, A re-examination of the structure of the mammalian liver II. The hepatic lobule and its relation to the vascular and biliary system. Amer. J. Anat. 85:379, 1949.

8. Rappaport AM, Borowy ZJ, Lougheed WM, Lotto WN, Subdivision of hexagonal liver lobules into a structural and functional unit; role in hepatic physiology and pathology. Anat. Rec. 119:11, 1954.

9. Rappaport AM, The structural and functional unit in the human liver (liver acinus). Anat. Rec. 130:673, 1958.

10. Rappaport AM, The microcirculatory hepatic units. Microvasc. Res. 6:212, 1973.

11. Grisham JW, Nopanitaya W, Compagno J, Scanning electron microscopy of the liver: a review of methods and results. In: Progress in liver diseases. Vol. V, Popper H, Schaffner F (eds), New York, Grune and Stratton, 1976, p.1.

12. Hampton JP, An electron microscope study of hepatic uptake and excretion of submicroscopic particles injected into the blood stream and into the bile duct. Acta Anat. 32:262, 1958.

13. Goresky CA, The transport and net removal of substances by the intact liver. In: The liver: quantitative aspects of structure and function, Baumgartner G, Preisig B (eds), Basle, S. Karger, 1973.

14. Segall HN, An experimental anatomical investigation of the blood and bile channels of the liver. Surg. Gynec. Obstet. 37:152, 1923.

15. Hjortsjö CH, The internal topography of the liver: studies by roentgen and injection technique. Nord. Med. 38:745, 1948.

16. Gillfillan RS, Anatomic study of the portal vein and its main branches. Arch. Surg. 61:449, 1950.

17. Elias H, Petty D, Cross anatomy of blood vessels and ducts within the human liver. Amer. J. Anat. 90:59, 1952.

18. Bradley SE, Ingelfinger FJ, Bradley GP, Curry JJ, The estimation of hepatic blood flow in man. J. clin. Invest. 24:890, 1945.

19. Caesar J, Shaldon S, Chiandussi L, Guevara L, Sherlock S, The use of indocyanine green in the measurement of hepatic blood flow and as a test of hepatic function. Clin. Sci. 21:43, 1961.

20. Rees JR, Redding VJ, Ashfield R, Hepatic blood-flow measurement with Xenon-133. Evidence for separate hepatic arterial and portal venous pathways. Lancet 2:562, 1964.

21. Neumayer AA, Problems of the hepatic circulation in health and disease. Gastroenterology 47:343, 1964.

22. Winkler K, Larsen JA, Munker T, Tygstrup N, Determination of hepatic blood flow in man by simultaneous use of five test substances in two parts of the liver. Scand. J. clin. Lab. Invest. 17:473, 1965.

23. Mackenzie RJ, Leiberman DP, Mathie GC, Rice GC, Harper AM, Blumgart LH, Liver blood flow measurement: the interpretation of Xenon-133 clearance curves. Acta chir. Scand. 142:519, 1976.

24. Ueda H, Circulation of hepatic artery and portal vein. In: Aktuelle Probleme der Hepatologie, Martini GA (ed), Stuttgart, Georg Thieme Verlag, 1962.

25. Pabst HW, Peller P, Behringer W, Isotopenstudien über die Leberdurchblutung und ihre Beeinflussbarkeit. Klin. Wschr. 40:505, 1962.

26. Novikoff AB, Essner E, The liver cell, some new approaches to its study. Amer. J. Med. 29:102, 1960.

27. Fawcett DW, Observations on the cytology and electron microscopy of hepatic cells. J. nat. Cancer Inst. 15:1475, 1955.

28. Cowdry EV, The mitochondrial constituents of protoplasm. Cargenie Inst. Washington, 271:39, 1918.

29. Altmann HW, Allgemeine morphologische Pathologie des Cytoplasmas. Die Pathobiosen. In: Handbuch der allgemeine Pathologie, Büchner F (ed), Berlin, Springer, 1955, p.419.

30. Manelidis EE, Pathological swelling and vacuolization of cells. In: Frontiers of cytology, Palay SL (ed), New Haven, Yale University Press, 1958, p.417.

31. Miller LL, Bale WF, Synthesis of all plasma protein fraction except gamma globulin by the liver. J. exp. Med. 99:125, 1954.

32. Porter KR, The submicroscopic morphology of protoplasm. Harvey Lect. 51:175, 1957.

33. Porter KR, Bruni G, An electron microscopic study of the early effects of 3'-Mc-DAB on rat liver cells. Cancer Res. 19:997, 1959.

34. Remmer H, Die Induktion Arzneimittel abbauender Enzyme im Endoplasmatisch Reticulum der Leberzelle durch Pharmaka. Dtsch. Med. Wschr. 92:2001, 1967.

35. Essner E, Novikoff AB, Human hepatocellular pigments and lysosomes J. Ultrastruct. Res. 3:374, 1960.

36. Palay S, The morphology of secretion. In: Frontiers of cytology, Palay SL, (ed), New Haven, Yale University Press. 1958, p.305.

37. Ellinger P, Hirt A, Mikroskopische Untersuchung an lebenden Organen; Methodik: Intravital Mikroskopie. Z. ges. Anat. (abt 1), 90:791, 1929.

38. White TT, Manometry and physiology of the bile ducts. In: Surgery of the liver, pancreas and biliary tract, Najarian J, Delaney J, (eds), New York, Stratton, 1975.

39. Daniel O, The value of radionanometry in bile duct surgery. Amer. Roy. Coll. Surg. Eng. 51:357, 1972.

40. Hand BH, Anatomy and function of the exhepatic biliary system. Clin. in gasteroenterology 2:3, 1973.

41. Hallenbeck GA, Biliary and pancreatic intraductal pressures. In: Handbook of Physiology, sect. 6, Vol. II, Code CF (ed), Washington DC, 1967, Amer. Phys. Soc. p. 1007.

42. Admirand W, Way LW, The gallbladder and pancreas. In: Gastro-intestinal disease, sect. 5, Sleisinger M, Fordtran J (eds), Philadelphia, Saunders, 1973, p. 352.

43. Ivy AC, Drewyek GE, Orndorff BH, The effect of cholecystokinin on human gallbladder. Amer. J. Physiol. 93:661, 1930.

44. Ostrow JD, Absorption by the gallbladder of bile salts; sulfobromphtalein and iodipamide. J. Lab. clin. Med. 74:482, 1969.

45. Wheeler HO, Concentration of the gallbladder. Amer. J. Med. 51:588, 1971.

46. Koster HA, Shapiro A, Lerner H, On the rate of secretion of bile. Amer. J. Physiol. 115:23, 1936.

47. Cameron R, Some problems of biliary cirrhosis. Brit. med. J. 1:535, 1958.

48. Brauer RW, Leong GF, Holloway RJ, The effect of perfusion, pressure and temperature on bile flow and bile secretion pressure. Amer. J. Physiol. 177:103, 1954.

49. Javitt NB, The cholestatic syndrome. Amer. J. Med. 51:637, 1971.

50. Sperber I, Biliary secretion of organic anions and its influence on bile flow. In: The biliary system. Taylor W (ed), Oxford, Blackwell, 1965.

51. Wheeler HO, Determinants of the flow and composition of bile. Gastro-enterology 40:584, 1961.

52. Hofmann AF, Alan F, The enterohepatic circulation of bile acids in man. In: Clinics in gasteroenterology, Vol. 6, no. 1, Baumgarter G (ed), Philadelphia Saunders, 1977.

53. Berge Henegouwen GP, van, Galzuren en cholestase, Thesis Nijmegen, 1974.

54. Grafflin AL, Excretion of fluorescein by liver in the normal and abnormal conditions in vivo, observed with fluorescent microscope. Amer. J. Anat. 81:63, 1947.

55. Mendeloff AJ, Fluorescence of intravenously administered Rose Bengal appears only in hepatic polygonal cells. Proc. Soc. exp. Biol. Med. 70:556, 1949.

56. Hanzon V, Liver cell secretion under normal and pathologic conditions studied by fluorescence microscopy on living rats. Acta physiol. Scand. 28 suppl. 101:1, 1952.

57. Boyer JL, Bloomer JR, Canalicular bile secretion in man. Studies utilizing the biliary clearance of (^{14}C) mannitol. J. clin. Invest. 54:773, 1974.

58. Cowen AE, Korman MG, Hofmann A, Thomas PJ, Plasma disappearance of radio-activity after i.v. injection of labeled bile acids In man. Gastroenterology 68:1567, 1975.

59. Schanker LS, Secretion of organis compounds in bile. In: Handbook of physio-logy, sect. 6, Code CF, Heidel W (eds), Washington, Physiol. Soc. 1968, p. 2433.

60. Smith RL, The biliary excretion and enterohepatic circulation of drugs and other organic compounds. In: Progress in Drug Research, Jucker E (ed), Basle, Birkhäuser, 1966, p. 299.

61. Sperber I, Secretion of organic anions in the formation of urine and bile. Pharmac. Rev. 11:109, 1959.

62. Cahili GF, jr, Ashmore J, Earle AS, Zottu S, Glucose penetration into the liver. Amer. J. Physiol. 192:491, 1958.

63. Schanker LS, Hogben C, Biliary excretion of inulin sucrose and mannitol: analysis of bile formation. Amer. J. Physiol. 200:1087, 1961.

64. Solomon HM, Schanker LS, Hepatic transport of organic cations: active uptake of a quaternary ammonium compound procain amide ethobromide by rat liver slices. Biochem. Pharmacol. 12:621, 1963.

65. Priestly BG, O'Reilly WJ, Protein binding and the excretion of some azo dyes in rat bile. J. Pharm. Pharmacol. 18:41, 1966.

66. Levi AJ, Gatmaitan Z, Arias IM, Two hepatic cytoplasmic protein fractions, Y and Z, and their possible role in the hepatic uptake of bilirubin, sulphobromophtalein and other anions. J. clin. Invest. 48:2156, 1969.

67. Schanker LS, Hepatic transport of organic cations. In: The biliary system, Taylor W (ed), Oxford, Blackwell, 1965 p. 469.

68. Staedeler F, Über die Farbstoffe der Galle. Justin Lubigs. Amer. Chem. 132:323, 1864.

69. Ehrlich P, Sulfodiazobenzol, ein Reagens auf Bilirubin. Zbl. Klin. Med. 45:721, 1883.

70. Hijmans van den Bergh AA, Muller P, Über eine direkte und einde indirekte Diazoreaktion auf Bilirubin. Biochem. Z. 77:90, 1916.

71. Cole PH, Lathe GH, The separation of serum pigments giving the direct and indirect Van den Berh reaction. J. clin. Path. 6:99, 1953.

72. Ostrow JD, The protein-binding of C-14 bilirubin in human and murin serum. J. clin. Invest. 42:1286, 1963.

73. Brandt KH, The bilirubin story. Folia med. neerl. 15:167, 1972.

74. Brown WR, Grodsky GM, Carbone J, Intracellular distribution of triated bilirubin during hepatic uptake and excretion. Amer. J. Physiol. 207:1237, 1965.

75. Butt HR, Foulk WT, Hoffmann HN, Bilirubin metabolism. In: Modern Trends in Gasteroenterology 3. Card WI (ed), London, Butterworths, 1961.

76. Fleischner G, Arias JM, Recent advances in bilirubin formation, transport, metabolism and excretion. Amer. J. Med. 49:576, 1970.

77. Hoffmann HN, II, Whitcomb FF, jr, Butt HR, Bollman JL, Bile pigments of jaundice. J. clin. Invest. 39:132, 1960.

78. Wheeler HO, Inorganic ions in bile. In: The biliary tract, Taylor W (ed), Oxford, Blackwell, 1965.

79. Moulin D, de, Geel en groen zien in het verleden. In: Pathologie van lever en galwegen. Bernards JA, Tongeren JHM (eds), Nijmegen, Thoben Offset, 1971.

80. Popper H, The pathogenesis of cholestasis. In: Surgery of the liver, pancreas and biliary tract, Natarisian J, Delaney J (eds), Grune and Stratton New York, 1975, p.391.

81. Sherlock S, In: Diseases of the liver and biliary system. Scientific Publication. London, Blackwell, 1975, p.1.

82. Popper H, The pathogenesis of cholestasis. Surgery of the liver, pancreas and biliary tract, p. 391, 1975.

83. Popper H, Szanlo PB, Intrahepatic cholestasis ("cholangitis"). Gastro-enterology 31:683, 1956.

84. Schaffner F, Popper H, Morphologic studies of cholestasis. Gastroenterology 37, p. 565, 1959.

85. Desmet VJ, Morphologic and histiochemical aspects of cholestasis. In: Progress of liver diseases, Vol.IV, Popper H, Schaffner F, (eds), New York, Grune and Stratton, 1972, p. 97.

86. Schalm L, De pathogenese van de verschillende vormen van icterus. In: Pathologie van lever en galwegen, Bernards JA, Tongeren JHM, Nijmegen, Thoben Offset, 1971, p. 117.

87. Schaffner F, Popper H, Classification and mechanism of cholestasis. In: Liver and biliary disease, Wright R, Alberti K, Karran S, Millward-Sadler GH, (eds), Saunders, London, 1979, p. 296.

88. Schersten T, Metabolic difference between hepatitis and cholestasis in human liver. In: Progress in liver diseases, Vol. IV, Popper H, Schaffner F, (eds), New York, Grune and Stratton, 1972, p. 133.

89. Ozawa K, Takasan H, Kitamora O, Alteration in liver mitochondrial metabolism in a patient with biliary obstruction due to liver carcinoma. Amer. J. Surg. 126:653, 1973.

90. Cameron R, Hou PG, Biliary cirrhosis. Oliver and Boyd (eds), Edinburgh, 1962.

2. IN VIVO NUCLEAR MEDICAL TECHNIQUES FOR THE EVALUATION OF LIVER FUNCTION

P.H. COX, H.S.L.M. TJEN

2.1. INTRODUCTION

Undoubtedly the most widely known in vivo nuclear medical technique for evaluating the liver is scintigraphy using radioactive colloids. The fact that intravenously injected colloidal particles accumulate in the phagocytes of the reticulo endothelial system and in particular the Kupffer cells of the liver has long been known. Voigt (1,2) first attempted quantitative studies of colloid biodistribution by measuring the distribution of silver colloid in rabbits using chemical and microscopic assays.

In 1937 Reeves and Morgan (3) reported on the first use of a colloid to visualize the liver phagocytes, thorotract, a radiocontrast medium and in 1947 Sheppard et al (4) paved the way for modern imaging techniques by introducing radiogold[198] colloid. This was first used for liver scintigraphy by Stirret (5) but because of its poor radiation characteristics it was later replaced by Technetium Sulphur colloid (6) although many other colloids have been used at one time or another (7).

Colloidal particles are removed from the blood by the phagocytic action of the Kupffer cells which form part of the reticulo-endothelial system and are uniformly distributed throughout the liver. By using this capacity a static image of the liver can be obtained using radioactive colloids which provides information about the localization, shape and size of the liver together with information concerning focal and diffuse abnormalities. However a study of the vast literature on the subject clearly demonstrates a considerable overlap in the criteria differentiating between normal variations, artefacts and abnormality. A number of variations in the size and shape of the normal liver have been described which form a limitation to the accuracy of the interpretation of scintigrams (8,9). The imprint of extrahepatic structures can also alter the liver shape (7,10). Overlap by other organs can cause reduction of count rates and treatments such as radiotherapy reduce accumulation of radioactivity in the

absence of true pathology. Objective criteria for abnormality are therefore
hard to define and the interpretation given to the images obtained is highly
subjective. The overall erroneous interpretation rate has been shown to vary
with the experience of the observer (11,12,13).

2.2. Liver scintigraphy and focal liver disease

A major indication for hepatic imaging is to distinguish between focal
defects and diffuse parenchymal disease. Space occupying lesions produce focal
defects; but on the other hand focal defects can occur in diffuse disease. The
reliability of hepatic imaging in focal disease is dependent on the size of the
lesion, its location in the liver and the sensitivity of the detector used
(14,15,16,17). Since focal defects may indicate a variety of pathological
conditions the specific nature of a local lesion can seldom be established by a
scintillation study alone. It has been suggested that more accurate information
about the nature of colloid filling defects in the liver can be provided by
multiple radionuclide studies (7,8,19, 20,21) or by using combined imaging
techniques (22,23). With these techniques an increase in diagnostic accuracy
has been claimed.

2.3. Liver scintigraphy and diffuse liver disease

Scintigraphic imaging is a diagnostic aid of limited value in diffuse
parenchymal liver disease. The sensitivity of detection of diffuse involvement
in mild disease states is less than observed with focal defects. These non-
specific findings vary from normal activity distribution, "patchy" or "mottled"
distribution within the liver, to focal defects (7,8,10,24). In cases of advanced cirrhosis a so called colloid shift to the reticulo-endothelial system
of spleen and bone marrow may occur. Antar (25) speaks of reticulo-endothelial
failure of the liver. The characteristic findings in such cases are decreased
radioactivity in the often enlarged liver, increased activity in an enlarged
spleen, increased accumulation of radioactivity in the bone marrow and high
radioactivity in the cardiac blood pool. All of this results from reduced
hepatic blood flow (26), a decrease in the hepatic clearance of the radiocolloid reflecting injury to the liver cells. In other diffuse liver diseases
such as acute or chronic hepatitis some of these findings may also occur (10,
27). DeNardo et al (28) reported the measurement of radiocolloid clearance
rates by liver and other reticulo-endothelial tissues as an aid to the differentiation between a number of diffuse liver diseases.

2.4. Accuracy of liver scintigraphy

The diagnostic value of liver scintigraphy is limited by the rate of occurence of false positive and negative results. Several investigations have eluated the accuracy of liver scan in focal disease in large series of patients (8,14,15,16,17,29,30). In 1977 De Ruiter et al (17) found an overall agreement rate of 83% when correlating scintigraphic to autopsy findings. These results are somewhat better than the accuracy rate reported by other investigators which vary from 77 - 80%. In De Ruiter's series false positive reports occurred in 15% and false negative reports in 18% of cases. In other investigations false positive reports vary between 9 - 30% and false negative reports between 12 to 15%. The observation of De Ruiter (17) that the accuracy of liver scintigraphy increases in the presence of an enlarged liver is worth mentioning. Covington (14,15) has discussed the errors and anomalies which may lead to false positive and false negative interpretations of scintigrams.

2.5. Liver scintigraphy and jaundice

Colloid scintigraphy of the liver in jaundiced patients provides only non-specific information and has therefore a limited diagnostic value. As in diffuse liver disease patterns of "reticulo-endothelial liver failure" can occur. Findings of focal lesions can be due to space-occupying lesions but may also be caused by dilated bile-ducts (8,10,19,31). A distinct defect or diminished iso-tope uptake in the region of the porta hepatis in jaundiced patients may be due to metastatic disease or anatomic variation but is also highly suspect for en-larged bile-ducts (32) and may indicate extrahepatic biliary obstruction. Heck (31) established criteria for the determination of biliary-duct enlargement and found an overall diagnostic reliability of 78%. In cases of obstructive jaundice in children caused by biliary atresia, choledochal cysts or the inspissated bile syndrome no distinguishing features could be observed (33,34). However in some cases the presence of liver disease was confirmed, but no definitive in-formation was provided as to the site of obstruction.

Several investigators compared the results obtained by nuclear liver imaging with those of ultrasound and CT-scanning (35,36,37,38,39,40). A similar degree of overall accuracy in diagnosing focal disease has been found for ultrasound (39), but both ultrasound and CT-scanning can differentiate space-occupying lesions with a higher degree of accuracy than scintigraphy. In diffuse liver disease, such as cirrhosis, nuclear imaging is superior but in general colloid scans seem to produce more false positive results in comparison to ultrasound and CT-scanning (38,39,41). In obstructive jaundice CT-scanning and ultrasound are of more value due to the demonstration of dilated intrahepatic bile-ducts. The combination of ultrasound and nuclear imaging more accurately assesses focal hepatic lesions than either modality alone (38,42). CT-hepatic imaging appears only occasionally to give extra information.

2.6. Cholescintigraphy, the functional study of liver and biliary tract

The concept that the functional capacity of the liver might be assessed by meassuring the ability of liver cells to remove and excrete an intravenously injected dye was first introduced in 1901 by Abel and Rowntree (43). In 1923 the first paper dealing with the use of Rose Bengal for the study of liver function was presented (44) The dye was administered intravenously in dogs and the rate of elimination from the blood stream and the influence of liver injury on the rate of elimination was estimated. The first results of the Rose Bengal test in human subjects was reported by the same investigator in 1924. The introduction of a radioactive Rose Bengal uptake excretion test by Taplin et al (45) in 1955 represented a further development of the earlier Rose Bengal test. A new era for studying liver function with radioactive substances was heralded by this development.

2.7. ^{131}I-Rose Bengal

Taplin et al (45) reported on the results of a study of the turnover of radioactive dye in rabbits to prove the potential clinical applicability in liver and biliary tract disease. A gamma ray scintillation counter and recording equipment were used to make external measurements over the liver area. In the same publication they also demonstrated the preliminary clinical results in patients with some common diseases of liver. These diseases seem to produce fairly typical uptake excretion patterns, which are readily distinguishable from those reported in normal individuals.

Rose Bengal is a fluorescein derivate and is labeled with ^{131}I, which emits both gamma and beta rays of several energies and has a half life of 8.14 days. It is removed from the blood exclusively by the polygonal cells of the liver and excreted via the bile. Peak levels in the liver are reached within 30 - 40 minutes after injection of the substance; normally it appears in the duodenum in 15 - 20 minutes (46) Meurman (47) studied the distribution and kinetics of ^{131}I-Rose Bengal in animals.

Among other things he described autoradiographic findings, which show that

[131]I-Rose Bengal is mainly taken up centrilobularly in the liver of normal animals. In necrotic areas of damaged livers a very high uptake of the substance was also shown. A notable fact is that when retention of ^{131}I-Rose Bengal occurs in the blood the radioactivity in different organs was usually increased, for exemple in the stomach wall. Therefore is it possible for the dye to be excreted in the gastro-intestinal tract, even when there is complete obstruction of the common bile-duct. Nordyke (48) also reviewed the metabolic and physiologic aspects of ^{131}I-Rose Bengal in studying liver function and the patency of the biliary tract and confirmed earlier findings of Meurman (47). Burke (49) first reported the use of the scintillation camera with ^{131}I-Rose Bengal for the continuous visualization of the dynamics of liver uptake and excretion.

2.8. Clinical application of ^{131}I-Rose Bengal

Following the introduction of the test by Taplin (45) various applications of the ^{131}I-Rose Bengal test have been described. "Liver counting" to estimate liver function is a relatively insensitive method to distinguigh between normal and abnormal function (50,51). The estimation of blood clearance is a more sensitive and less complex alternative technique (52,53).

The first application of the test in relation to jaundice was reported by Eyler et al (54). Since then several similar publications have appeared. Winston and Blahd (54) reviewed the results of several investigators who used rectilinear scanners and scintillation cameras. They pointed out that with this tracer study several conclusions about the etiology of jaundice can be drawn, but that the differentiation of partial biliary tract obstruction and cholestasis is not reliable. Several modifications to the test and a detailed study of the results could not significantly increase the reliability of the test in relation to the differential diagnosis or the site of obstruction (46,48,56,57, 58). The test has made a significant contribution to the difficult differential diagnosis of jaundice in childhood (59,60,61. For the diagnosis of choledochal cysts the test has also proved to be a most effective procedure (62,63,64). Shoop (65) reported a cirrhotic patient with hepatoma in whom the tumour concentrated the tracer as well or better than the remaining fibrotic liver tissue. Leakage of bile into the peritoneal cavity due to trauma or biopsy can also be detected (61,66). Eikman (67) used the test to study the patency of the cystic duct as an diagnostic aid in acute cholecystitis.

The disadvantages of the ^{131}I-Rose Bengal limit its wide spread use as a radiopharmaceutical. [131]Iodine has physical properties which are not optimal for imaging and which lead to relatively high radiation doses. The thyroid must be blocked before starting the study and there is a relative high rate of false positive reports (53). Other labeled agents have also been tested and used for clinical investigations. Reports have appeared about ^{131}I-Toluidine blue (68), ^{123}I-Bronsulphalein (69), ^{123}I-Indocyanine green (70), ^{131}I-Asialo-orosomucoid (71), and ^{111}In-phenolphtalein (72).

2.9. Tc^{99m}-labeled hepato biliary agents

Scintigraphic imaging of the hepato biliary system has significantly improved with development of Tc^{99m}-labeled reagents. These radiopharmaceuticals do not have the disadvantages of the ^{131}I-labeled agents and the excellent physical characteristics of Tc^{99m} make them preferable for organ imaging. Many complexes labeled with Technetium have been proposed as hepato biliary agents since the first report from Baker et al (79) about their findings with Tc^{99m}-Pyridoxylideneglutamate (Tc^{99m}-PDG) as cholescintigraphic agent (73,74,75, 76,77,78). A number of Tc^{99m}-labeled amino acid complexes of Pyridoxylidene showed excellent hepato biliary excretion and found therefore a wide application in the clinical investigation of hepato biliary disorders (74,79,80,81,82,83,84, 85). Since 1976 hepato biliary imaging with derivatives of iminodiacetic acid (Ida) have been performed and the first clinical reports seem again to indicate improvement (78,86,87,88).

2.10. Tc^{99m}-Pyridoxilideneglutamate

In 1975 in an extensive investigation Baker et al (79) reported the experimental aspects and clinical applicability of Tc^{99m}-PDG. The compound showed a high rapid concentration in the polygonal liver cells with a good visualization of the liver 3 - 5 minutes post injection and of the gall-bladder about 10 minutes after injection.

Good experimental work on this subject was also done by Fotopoulos (81) and Jenner (75). They confirmed earlier statements that pyridoxal complexes are valuable in the diagnosis of disturbances of the hepato biliary tract, and that the study is a useful supplement to radiocontrast studies. Ronai et al (74) reported on the clinical findings with Tc^{99m}-PDG in 70 patients; they described the distribution patterns in normal subjects, patients suffering from right upper quadrant abdominal pain and jaundiced patients. The normal findings included a visualization of the biliary tract and the gall-bladder within 10 - 15 minutes and accumulation in the gastro-intestinal tract within 20 minutes.

2.11.Tc^{99m}-PDG test in gall-bladder disease

In the investigation of abdominal pain, Ronai (74) found the cholescintigram a reliable investigation to detect acute inflammatory disease of gall-
bladder. However in most cases of chronic cholecystitis a normal cholescintigram was found. In all patients there was a similarity with X-ray investigation.
Poulose (80) found no visualisation of the gall-bladder in patients with
chronic cholecystitis, but used the Tc^{99m}-PDG scan in patients when focal
defects in or near the usual gall-bladder bed were found on the colloid scan.
When the defects fill in on the Tc^{99m}-PDG scan it confirms that they were
secondary to the gall-bladder impression or to a partial intrahepatic gall-
bladder and were not due to metastases. Stadalnik et al (89) reported a 100%
accuracy of the Tc^{99m}-PDG scan in cholecystitis and compared the results with
cholecystography and ultra sonography. A normal gall-bladder can fail to accumulate radioactivity (90,91).

2.12.Tc^{99m}-PDG test in jaundice

The problem of finding reliable parameters to determine whether the cause
of jaundice is intra or extra hepatic has also constituted a challenge for cholescintigraphy. Several attempts where made to modify or extend the original
Tc^{99m}-PDG test for more accuracy in differentiating between medical and surgical jaundice (74,80,82,83,85). The complete obstruction pattern generally posed
no great problem, on the contrary the patterns of partial obstruction or delayed excretion on the sequential scintigrams potentiated difficulties of differential diagnosis. In the study of Ronai (74) in 36 jaundiced patients, the
absence of gastro-intestinal activity at 18 hours after injection of the radio-
pharmacon allowed a reliable diagnosis of complete extra biliary obstruction.
Further evidence supporting this diagnosis was provided by presence of a defect
in the liver or back-ground activity due to the presence of the distended gall-
bladder. Ronai (74) distinguished a negative gall-bladder image, a so called
Courvoisier sign from a non-visualized gall-bladder. He found this typical
phenomenon In 80% in patients with biliary obstruction. In patients with incomplete biliary obstruction there is delayed excretion of the reagent into the
gastro-intestinal tract. Hepato cellular disease may also give this pattern.
Ronai (74) stated that an incomplete biliary obstruction is difficult to differentiate from a liver parenchyma disturbance unless a scintigraphic Courvoisier
sign or distended common bile-duct is seen in the scintigram. Verdegaal (83)
also used the Courvoisier sign in the differentiation between intra and extra

hepatic jaundice, combined with the results of ultrasound. Lubin (85) approach-
ed the problem of distinguishing between hepato cellular disease and obstructive jaundice by estimating the time of appearence in the intestine and by
using the 20 minutes/5 minutes ratio as a measure of clearance efficiency of
the polygonal cell. He also related this appearance time to bilirubin values
and found a delayed excretion of the agent (30 - 180 minutes after injection)
at a bilirubin level of 2.8 mg%, a very delayed (24 hours) excretion by a
bilirubin value of 11 mg% and no visualization at a bilirubin of 12.2 mg%. However his overall accuracy in this series patients was reported as 72.4%.
Poulose (80) showed less optimism in his report and regarded the Tc^{99m}-PDG test
as less helpful to distinguish intra hepatic and extra hepatic jaundice. Some
other indications for the use of Tc^{99m}-labeled components are assessing the
patency of a biliary intestinal anastomosis, assessing functional disturbances
of the sphincter of Oddi (82) and demonstrating intra peritoneal bile-leakage
(81).

2.13. Technetium-Ida derivatives

Although reports of further developments of pyridoxylene derivatives still
appear in the literature there is little doubt that the introduction of iminodiacetic acid derivatives by Loberg in 1976 led to the more or less exclusive
use of these reagents in the ensueing years. Since 1976 more than 150 publications have appeared on the use of Ida-derivatives which is some measure of
their rapid acceptance as the reagents of choice for liver function studies.
Much of the available experience will be discussed in ensueing chapters and
therefore will not be reviewed here.

REFERENCES

1. Voigt J, Untersuchungen über die Verteilung und das Schicksal des Kolloiden Silbers im Säugetierkörper. I. Biochem. Z. 62:280, 1914.

2. Voigt J, Untersuchungen über die Verteilung und das Schicksal des Kolloiden Silbers im Säugetierkörper. II. Biochem. Z. 63:409, 1914.

3. Reaves RJ, Morgan JE, The retention of Thorium dioxide by the reticulo endothelial system. Radiology 29:612, 1937.

4. Sheppard CW et al, Studies of the distribution of intravenously administered colloidal sols of manganese dioxide and gold in human beings and dogs using radioisotopes. J. Lab. clin. Med. 32:274, 1947.

5. Stirett LA, Yuhl ET, Cassen B, Clinical application of hepatic radioactivity surveys. Amer. J. Gasteroent. 21:310, 1954.

6. Nelp WB, An evaluation of colloids for RES function studies. In: Radiopharmaceuticals, Subramanian G et al (eds), New York, Society of Nuclear Medicine, p.349, 1975.

7. Jonsson K, Wallace S et al, The use of prostaglandin E for enhanced visualization of the splanclinic circulation, Radiology 125:373, 1975.

8. McAfee JG, Ause RG, Wagner HN, Diagnostic value of scintillation scanning of the liver. Arch. intern. Med. 116:95, 1965.

9. Mould RF, An investigation of variations in normal liver shape. Brit. J. Radiol. 45:486, 1972.

10. Berghuis PHE, Een scintigrafisch onderzoek van morfologie en functie van de lever. Ph.D. Thesis, University of Rotterdam, 1976.

11. Ludbrook J, Slavotinek AH, Ronai PM, Observer error in reporting on liver scans for space-occupying lesions. Gastroenterology 62:1013, 1972.

12. Conn HA, Spencer RP, Observer error in liver scans. Gasteroenterology 62:1085, 1972.

13. Nishiyama H et al, Interpretation of liver images. J. nucl. Med. 16:11, 1975.

14. Covington EE, Pitfalls in liver photoscan. Amer. J. Roentgenol. 109:745, 1970.

15. Covington EE, The accuracy of liver photoscans. Amer. J. Roentgenol. 109:742, 1970.

16. Lunia S, Parthasarathy KL, Bakshi S, Bender MA, An evaluation of ^{99m}Tc-sulfur colloid liver scintiscans and their usefulness in metastatic workup: a review of 1,424 studies. J. nucl. Med. 16:62, 1975.

17. Ruiter DJ, Byck W, Pauwels EKJ, Taconis WK, Spaander PJ, Correlation of scintigraphy with short interval autopsy in malignant focal liver disease. A study of 59 cases. Cancer 39:172, 1977.

18. Muroff LR, Johnson PM, The use of multiple radionuclide imaging to differentiate the focal intrahepatic lesion. Amer. J. Roentgenol. 121:728, 1974.

19. Shtasel P, Liver and spleen. In: Speak to me in nuclear medicine. Shtasel P (ed), New York, London, Harper and Row, 1976.

20. Yeh SOJ, Leeper RD, Benua RS. A study of filling defect in the liver and spleen with multiple radionuclides. Clin. Bull. 7:1, 1977.

21. Yeh SH, Liu OK, Huang MJ, Technetium-99m-pyridoxylideneglutamate (Tc-99m-PG) sequential scintiphotography in the detection of intrahepatic stones. J. nucl. Med. 18:635, 1977.

22. Taylor KJW, Grey scale ultrasound imaging. Radiology 119:445, 1977.

23. Gooneratne NS, Quinn JL, Hepatic left lobe lesions. Clinical usefulness of multiple imaging techniques to increase lesion detectability. Clin. nucl. Med. 2:377, 1977.

24. Ephraim KH, Nucleaire Geneeskunde. Ned. Bibliotheek der Geneeskunde, nr. 68, Leiden, Stafleu, 1972.

25. Antar MA, Szitlal JJ, Spencer RP, Liver imaging during reticuloendothelial failure. Clin. nucl. Med. 9:293, 1977.

26. Shaldon S, Chiandussi L, Guevara L, Caesar J, Sherlock S, The measurement of hepatic blood flow and intrahepatic shunted blood flow by colloidal heat-denatured human serum albumin labelled with I^{131}. J. clin. Invest. 40:1346, 1961.

27. Luthra HS, Scherl ND, Golden D, Finkel M, Collica CJ, Scintiphotography in hepatitis. Arch. intern. Med. 122:207, 1968.

28. DeNardo SJ, Diagnosis of cirrhosis and hepatitis by quantitative hepatic and other reticuloendothelial clearance rates. J. nucl. Med. 17:449, 1976.

29. Marty W, Schwarz H, Die Stellung der Scintigraphischen Beurteilung der metastasen Leber. Helv. chir. Acta 44:499, 1977.

30. Cedermark BJ, Schultz SS, Bakshi S, Parthasarathy KL, Mittelman A, Evans JT, The value of liver scan in the follow-up study of patients with adenocarcinoma of the colon and rectum. Surg. Gynec. Obstet. 144:745, 1977.

31. Heck L, Gottschalk A, The appearance of intrahepatic biliary duct dilatation on the liver scan. Radiology, 99:135, 1971.

32. Drum DE, Christacopoulos JS, Hepatic scintigraphy in clinical decision making. J. nucl. Med. 13:908, 1972.

33. Dacosta H, Ghandi R, Deshmukh S, Puri K, Loken M, Hepatosplenic scintigraphy in children with obstructive jaundice. Clin. nucl. Med. 2:381, 1977.

34. Smith AL, Mowat AP, Williams R, Hepatic scintigraphy in managament of infants and children with liver disease. Arch. Dis. Childh. 52:633, 1977.

35. Jääskelainen I, Rissanen P, Comparison of ultrasound and isotope scannings in detection of liver metastases. Scan. J. clin. Lab. Invest. 108:87, 1969.

36. Leyton B, Halpern S, Leopold G, Hagen S, Correlation of ultrasound and colloid scintiscan studies of the normal and diseased liver. J. nucl. Med. 14:27, 1973.

37. Taylor KJW, Carpenter DA, McCready VR, Ultrasound and scintigraphy in the differential diagnosis of obstructive jaundice. J. Clin. Ultrasound 2:105, 1974.

38. McCarthy CF, Davies ER, Wells PMT, A comparison of ultrasonic and isotope scanning in the diagnosis of liver disease. Brit. J. Radiol. 43:100, 1970.

39. Rasmussen SN, Hviid T, Mouridsen H, Petersen, The diagnosis of liver-metastases by ultrasonic and radioisotope scanning. Dan. med. Bull. 25:60, 1978.

40. Scherer U, Büll U, Rothe R, Eisenberg J, Schildberg FW, Meister P, Lissner J, Computerized tomography and nuclear imaging of the liver. A comparative study in 83 cases. Eur. J. Nucl. Med. 3:71, 1978.

41. Taylor KJW, Grey-scale ultrasound imaging. Radiology 119:445, 1977.

42. Grossman ZD, Comparison of nuclear imaging, gray scale ultra sonography and computed axial tomography of the liver. J. nucl. Med. 17:544, 1976.

43. Abel JJ, Rowntree LG, On the pharmacological action of some phtaleins and their derivatives with especial reference to their behaviour as purgatives. I. J. Pharmac. exp. Ther. 1:233, 1901.

44. Delprat GD jr, Studies on liver function; Rose Bengal elimination from blood as influenced by liver injury. Arch. intern. Med. 32:401, 1923.

45. Taplin G. Meridith M, jr, Kade H, The radioactive (^{131}I-tagged) Rose Bengal uptake-excretion test for liver function using external Gamma-ray scintillation counting technique. J. Lab. clin. Med. 5:665, 1955.

46. Neibling HA, Use of ^{131}I-Rose Bengal scans in diagnosis of biliary construction. Amer. Surg. 38:328, 1972.

47. Meurman L, On the distribution and kinetics of injected ^{131}I-Rose Bengal. Acta med. scand. 354:7, 1960.

48. Nordyke RA, Biliary tract obstruction and localisation with ^{131}I-Rose Bengal. Amer. J. Gastroent. 33:563, 1960.

49. Burke G, Halko A, Dynamic clinical studies with radioisotopes and the scintillation camera. Rose Bengal I-131 liver function studies. Jama Vol. 198, 6:140, 1966.

50. Rosenberg CA, Lee ND, Martignoni P, The use of radioactive Rose Bengal as a liver function test. Clin. Res. 4:39, 1956.

51. Moertel CG, Owen CA, Evaluation of the radioactive (^{131}I-tagged) Rose Bengal liver function test in non-jaundiced patients. J. Lab. clin. Med. 52:902, 1958.

52. Sapirstein LA, Simpson AM, Plasma clearance of Rose Bengal (tetra-iodo-brom-fluorescein). Amer. J. Physiol. 182:337, 1955.

53. Davies ER, Morris JN, Read AE, Powell N, ^{131}I-Rose Bengal scanning and clearance ratios in the investigation of jaundiced patients. Clin. Radiol. 27:227, 1976.

54. Eyler WR, Schuman BM, du Sault LA, Hinson RE, The radioiodinated Rose Bengal liver scans as an aid in the differential diagnosis of jaundice. Amer. J. Roentgenol. 84:469, 1965.

55. Winston MA, Blahd WH, ^{131}I-Rose Bengal imaging techniques in differential diagnosis of jaundiced patients. Sem. Nucl. Med. 2:167, 1972.

56. Whiting EG, Nusynowitz ML, Radioiodinated Rose Bengal testing in differential diagnosis of jaundice. Surg. Gynec. Obstet. 129:729, 1968.

57. Berk JE, Kawaguchi M, Soble AR, Goldstein SE, Differential diagnosis of jaundice: modified I^{131}-labeled Rose Bengal test. Arch. intern. Med. 111: 323, 1963.

58. Gamlen TR, Triger DR, Ackery DM, Fleming JS, Grant RW, Kenny RW, Maciver AG, Wright R, Quantitative liver imaging using ^{131}I-Rose Bengal as an index of liver function and prognosis. Gut 16:738, 1975.

59. Sharp HL, Krivit W, Lowman ST, The diagnosis of complete obstruction with Rose Bengal I[131]. J. Pediat. 70:46, 1967.

60. Thaler MM, Gellis SG, Studies in neonatal hepatitis and biliary atresia. Amer. J. Dis. Child. 116:280, 1968.

61. Rosenthall L, The application of radioiodinated Rose Bengal and colloidal radiogold in the detection of hepatobiliary disease. Green, St. Louis, 1969.

62. Williams LE, Fisher JH, Coutney RA, Preoperative diagnosis of choledochal-cyst by hepatoscintigraphy. New Eng. J. Med. 283:85, 1970.

63. Park CH, Garafola JH, O'Hara AE, Preoperative diagnosis of asymptomatic choledochal cyst by Rose Bengal liver scan. J. nucl. Med. 15:310, 1974.

64. Oshiumi Y, Nakayama Ch, Morita K, Numaguchi Y, Koga I, Matsuura K, Serial scintigraphy of choledochal cysts using ^{131}I-Rose Bengal and ^{131}I-Brom-sulphalein. Amer. J. Roentgenol. 128:796, 1977.

65. Shoop JD, Functional hepatoma demonstrated with Rose Bengal scanning. Amer. J. Roentgenol. 107:51, 1969.

66. Spencer RP, Kaplan MM, Glenn WW, Use of ^{131}I-Rose Bengal to follow bile leakage. Amer. J. dig. Dis. 12:1169, 1967.

67. Eikman EA, Cameron JL, Colman M, Natarajan TK, Dugal P, Wagner HN, A test for patency of the cystic duct in acute cholecystitis. Ann. intern. Med. 82:318, 1975.

68. Chen-Stute A, Chen T, Eickenbush W, ^{131}I-RTB-Methode zur Differenzierung von Leber- und Gallenwegserkrankungen. In: Nuklearmedizin. 15. Internatio-nale Jahrestagung der Gesellschaft für Nuklearmedizin, September 1977, Groningen. Schmidt HAE, Woldring M (eds), Stuttgart, Schattauer p. 581, 1978.

69. Goris M, I-iodo-bromsulphalein as a liver and biliary scanning agent. J. nucl. Med. 14:820, 1973.

70. Ansari AN, Atkins HL, Lambrecht RM, ^{123}I-indocyanin green as an agent for dynamic studies of the hepatobiliary system. In: Proceedings of a symposium on Dynamic Studies with Radioisotopes in Clinical Medicine and Research held by the IAEA in Knoxville, Tennessee, July 1974, Vol.I, Vienna IAEA, 1975.

71. Van Rijk PP, Purification, labelling and clinical applicability of radio-active asialo-orosomucoid. Ph.D. Thesis University of Utrecht, 1977.

72. Lin MS, ^{111}In-phenolphtalexon, a new chelate for extended cholescintigraphy: Formulation and preclinical characterization. Radiology 123:783, 1977.

73. Lin TH, Khentigan A, Winchell H, A ^{99m}Tc-labelled replacement for ^{131}I-Rose Bengal in liver and biliary tract studies. J. nucl. Med. 15:613, 1974.

74. Ronai PM, Baker RJ, Bellen JC, Technetium-99m-pyridoxylideneglutamate, a new hepatobiliary radiopharmaceutical. II clinical aspects. J. nucl. Med. 16:728, 1975.

75. Jenner RE, Clarke MB, Howard ER, Liver and gall-bladder imaging with Tech-netium-99m-dihydrothioctic acid and Technetium-99m pyridoxylideneglutamate - a study in the young pig. Brit. J. Radiol. 49:852, 1976.

76. Fritzberg AR, Lyster DM, Dolphin DH, ^{99m}Tc-Bioquin-7CA, a potential new hepatobiliary scanning agent. J. nucl. Med. 17:907, 1976.

77. Noronka OPA, Sewatkar AB, Ganatra RD, The transport, hepatobiliary distribution and clearance of ^{99m}Tc-Sn-Lidocaine Iminodiacetic acid, ^{99m}Tc-Sn-Lida. Int. J. Nucl. Med. Biol. 4:122, 1977.

78. Wistow BW, Subramanian G, Van Heertum RL, Henderson RW, Gagne GM, Hall RC, McAfee JG, An evaluation of ^{99m}Tc-labelled hepatobiliary agents. J. nucl. Med. 18:455, 1977.

79. Baker RJ, Bellen JC, Ronai PM, ^{99m}Tc- pyridoxylideneglutamate: a new rapid cholescintigraphic agent. J. nucl. Med. 15:476, 1974.

80. Poulose KP, Eckelman WC, Reba RC, Evaluation of ^{99m}Tc-pyridoxylideneglutamate for the differential diagnosis of jaundice. Clin. Nucl. Med. 1:70, 1976.

81. Fotopoulos A, Evaluation of Tc-99m-pyridoxalphenylalanine as a hepatobiliary imaging agent. Part. I. Experimental studies. J. nucl. Med. 18:1189, 1977.

82. Papadimitriou A, Fotopoulos C, Koutoulidis C, Chiotelis E, Tountas C, Evaluation of Tc-99m pyridoxalphenylalanine as a hepatobiliary agent. Part. II. Clinical tests. J. nucl. Med. 18:1194, 1977.

83. Verdegaal W, Esseveld M, Frensdorp E, Kruyswijk H, Warnus P, Winter WW, Yap-Tjok, Eerste ervaringen met ^{99m}Tc-pyridoxylideen-glutamaat. Ned. T. Geneesk. 121:1866, 1977.

84. Clarke DN, Brunt PW, Dascombe G, Macdonald AF, Mowat NAG, Sharp PF, Clinical value of ^{99m}Technetium pyridoxylideneglutamate for hepato-biliary imaging. In: Proceedings of the European Society of Nuclear Medicine, 2nd Congress on Nuclear Medicine, London (abstract) p.32, 1978.

85. Lubin E, Rachima M, Oren V, Weininger J, Trumper J, Kozenitzky I, Rechnic Y, Tc-99m-pyridoxylideneglutamate in jaundiced patients. J. nucl. Med. 19:24, 1978.

86. Tjen HSLM, Cox PH, Van der Pompe WB, Technetium-99m-labelled diethyl-acetanilido-imminodiacetate: a new hepatobiliary agent. A preliminary report. Brit. J. Rad. 50:735, 1977.

87. Rosenthall L, Shaffer EA, Lisbona R, Pare P, Diagnosis of hepatobiliary disease by ^{99m}Tc-Hida cholescintigraphy. Radiology 126:467, 1978.

88. Chiotellis E, Sawas-Dimopoulou G, Koutouliois C, Constantinides M, ^{99m}Tc-Hida a gall-bladder imaging agent. Experimental aspects. Eur. J. Nucl. Med. 3:41, 1978.

89. Stadalnik RC, Krauss JF, Matolo NM, Krohn KA, Evaluation of Tc-99m-pyridoxylideneglutamate cholescintigraphy as a diagnostic test for cholecystitis. J. nucl. Med. 18:635, 1977.

90. Eikman EA, Cameron JL, Colman M, Natarajan TK, Dugal P, Wagner HN, A test for patency of the cystic duct in acute cholecystitis. Ann. Int. Med. 82:318, 1975.

91. Ronai PM, Hepatobiliary radiopharmaceuticals: defining their clinical role will be a galling experience. J. nucl. Med. 18:488, 1977.

3. THE CHEMISTRY AND PHARMACY OF IDA-DERIVATIVES

P.H. COX

3.1. INTRODUCTION

The ideal radiopharmaceutical for hepatobiliary investigations should be
rapidly extracted from the blood by the hepatocytes following intravenous injection, pass rapidly through the hepatocytes and concentrate in the bile.
There should be little or no reabsorption from the intestinal tract and
minimal excretion in the urine. The labeling yield (with Tc^{99m}) should be high
and the product should be formulated as a sterile, pyrogen free one step labeling kit (1). The N-substituted iminodiacetic acid derivatives suggested by
Loberg in 1976 (2) fulfil many of these requirements.

3.2. Iminodiacetic acid derivatives

Iminodiacetic acid (fig. 1) is a well known organic compound used as an
intermediate in the synthesis of surfactants, chelating agents and complex
organic molecules. It is known to form complexes with heavy metals and as such
is a good candidate for combining with Tc^{99m}.

Lidocaine (fig. 2) is a widely used local anaesthetic which was first introduced into clinical patients in 1948. It is metabolized in the liver by
Dealkylation to Monoethylglycine and Xylidide. The latter is further metabolized
to 4 hydroxy-2-6-dimethylaniline which is excreted for 75% in the urine.

The N-acetanilido-iminodiacetic acid derivatives proposed by Loberg (2)
bear a structural resemblance to Lidocaine and as such are also rapidly accumulated in the hepatocytes. The chelating effect of the Ida present makes these
compounds amenable to complex formation with reduced Technetium. The basic structure of a number of clinically evaluated derivatives are shown in fig. 3.

The biological behaviour of Ida-derivatives does not however parallel that
of Lidocaine with the exception that they accumulate in the hepatocytes. Unlike
Lidocaine Ida-derivatives are not broken down in the hepatocytes but are excreted into the bile. The small amount of activity excreted via the kidneys is
extracted directly from the blood and the amount excreted is related to the

rapidity of clearance into the liver. Thus with hepatocyte malfunction the slow blood clearance is reflected as increased urinary excretion. It is thought that Ida-derivatives are excreted unchanged in the bile although this has been difficult to prove. Subramanian (3) reinjected bile containing Diethyl-Ida into rats and saw an unchanged biological distribution pattern from which he concluded that the Diethyl-Ida was present as free complex in the bile. In our laboratories however analysis of human bile samples suggested that Diethyl-Ida is bound to one or more bile salts. That this can occur was confirmed by incubating Tc^{99m}-diethyl-Ida with bile to demonstrate complex formation. It is not clear therefore whether complexation with bile salts occurs intracellularly or in the bile after excretion.

Contrary to Lidocaine it was also demonstrated that Diethyl-Ida was not reabsorbed from the intestine in animals (4) or humans (5).

3.3. The chemistry of Diethyl-Ida

It is clearly evident that whilst N-substituted-Ida-derivatives bear a chemical resemblance to Lidocaine their biological behaviour differs and therefore it is now pertinent to consider the chemistry of the Technetium-Ida complex.

In view of the widespread use of Diethyl-Ida it is not surprising that the bulk of the literature refers to this compound but this data is also relevant to other derivatives. ^{99m}Tc is eluated from the generator in the form of the Pertechnetate ion and in order to bind it to pharmacologically active carriers it is necessary to reduce it to a lower valency from usually TcIV or TcV. At the time that the first studies were made with Ida-derivatives the use of stannous chloride as a reducing agent was already well established, particularly in the formulation of instant labeling kits. It is therefore hardly surprising that this procedure was followed in the case of the Ida-derivatives.

With Technetium chelates used for bone, brain or kidney-scintigraphy it has generally been accepted that the Technetium is present in the IV or V valency state but some confusion has arisen as to whether the stannous ion was also incorporated into the complex or not.

3.4. The structure of Ida-complexes

Loberg (2) assigned a structure in which reduced Technetium was bound to the iminonitrogen group of Dimethyl-Ida and suggested that two molecules of Dimethyl-Ida formed a stable complex with TcIV. The fate of the tin was not

discussed further. On the basis of chromatographic studies Fonda and Pedersen
(6) confirmed Lobergs prognosis and suggested that in the case of Diethyl-Ida
the biscomplex formation proceded via the initial formation of a monocomplex
which could be seen as a double peak on the chromatogram. This double peak was
also observed by Cox and Tjen (7) and recent high performance liquid chromatography studies of Diethyl-Ida have confirmed the presence of two components
although variable in different formulations (8).

Loberg and Fields (9) confirmed the structure of Dimethyl-Ida-complex to be
two Ida-molecules bound to a TcIII ion via the nitrogen and oxygen atoms. This
structure does not include stannous ions the implication being that the tin
functions merely as an electron donor but is not incorporated into the complex.
It has since been confirmed that stannous ions are not incorporated into Technetium MDP or Glucoheptonate-complexes (11).

A further confirmation of this work was provided by the preparation of
Tc^{99m}-Diethyl-Ida using insoluble tin as a solid phase reducing agent, (12,13),
as well as with other insoluble reductants all of which function as electron
donors.

At the present time therefore it would appear to be safe to conclude that
the structure of Diethyl-Ida-complex is as shown in fig. 4 and that a percentage
of monomer is also present.

3.5. The quality control of Ida-derivatives

A number of Ida-derivatives are available for clinical use in the form of
freeze dried stannous labeling kits. Whilst stable for long periods of time it
is advisable to store vials at 0 - 4°C. Dimethyl-, p-isopropyl-, Diethyl- and
p-butyl-derivatives are all routinely available but of these the Diethyl is the
most widely used and is generally regarded as being the reagent of choice.

Labeling is performed by the aseptic addition of Pertechnetate eluate to
the labeling vial. The contents of the vial dissolve rapidly to form a colour-
less solution free of particles. The labeling of Diethyl-Ida is virtually in-
stantaneous but it is normally advised to wait 5 to 10 minutes after addition
of the Pertechnetate before use. The labeling of Dimethyl-Ida on the other hand
may not be complete for up to 30 minutes after reconstitution. Diethyl-Ida
injection consists of a mixture of Tc^{99m}-Diethyl-Ida, physiological saline and
stannous chloride. Possible impurities are free Pertechnetate, reduced Technetium hydroxide (which behaves as a colloid) and oxidized tin compounds which
may react with Technetium to form colloidal particles. As has already been

discussed the Tc^{99m}-diethyl-Ida (or other derivatives) may be present to varying amounts as monomer and dimer complexes but this does not appear to affect
the biological behaviour.

The quality control procedures therefore are primarily designed to detect
the presence of colloidal Technetium and free Pertechnetate in the presence of
the labeled compound. The simplest and most commonly used technique is thin
layer chromatography.

3.6. Thin layer chromatography

In our experience a simple thin layer chromatogram using silica gel as the
stationary phase and physiological saline as the continuous phase is a suitable
control procedure with Pertechnetate and Technetium colloid as control substances (4). In this system Tc^{99m}-diethyl-ida has an Rf value of 0.61, Pertechnetate 0.83 and colloid remains on the start line. In the case of Diethyl-Ida
labeling yields averaging 93.4% are routinely obtained and the amount of the
Pertechnetate present is less than 1%. Fig. 5 shows typical profile scans of
thin layer chromatograms of colloid, TcO$_4$ and Diethyl-Ida prepared with a
Berthold thin layer chromatography scanner. Alternatively electrophoresis gel
chromatography and high performance liquid chromatography have been proposed as
techniques for screening Ida-derivatives. Some recommended procedures are listed
below.

source (see references)	derivative	method
(14)	Dimethyl, Diethyl, Butyl-phenyl	(1) paper electrophoresis Whatman no 1 paper 0.05 M Phosphate buffer, pH 6.8 (2) paper electrophoresis Whatman 541 in Phosphate buffer pH 7.0
(15)	Diethyl	descending paper chromatography, Whatman no 1 using EDTA buffer or physiological saline
(6) (16)	Diethyl	gel chromatography Sephadex G 15
(17)	Dimethyl	(1) paper chromatography with 0.9% Sodium chloride (2) paper chromatography with Butanol:acid: water

source	derivative	method
		(3) paper chromatography in Acetonitrile: water
		(4) thin layer chromatography with 0.9% Sodium chloride
		(5) gel chromatography Sephadex G 25 in Sodium chloride Phosphate buffer
		(6) electrophoresis paper with Phosphate buffer
		(7) HPLC μ Bondapak C 18 column Acetonitrile Phosphate buffer
(18)	various derivates	(1) silica gel TLC strips (2) paper
(19)	various	HPLC

3.7. The stability of Tc^{99m}-Ida-derivates

In general Tc^{99m}-Ida-derivates are stable in vitro for long periods after labeling. Zivanovic et al (20) studied Tc^{99m}-Dimethyl-Ida and found it to be stable for more than 10 hours after reconstitution. Comparative studies in rat and man confirmed a similar stability in vivo. Tc^{99m}-Diethyl-Ida shows 95% labeling in vitro at 6 hours after reconstitution and biodistribution data confirms this stability in vivo (21). Contrary to the general experience with Technetium preparations the label shows an extreme stability under in vivo conditions which is reflected by the low secondary uptake in the thyroid and stomach even several hours post injection.

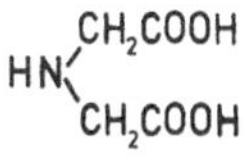

Fig. 1. Iminodiacetic acid (Ida).

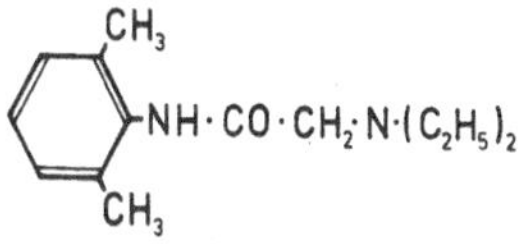

Fig. 2. Lidocaine.

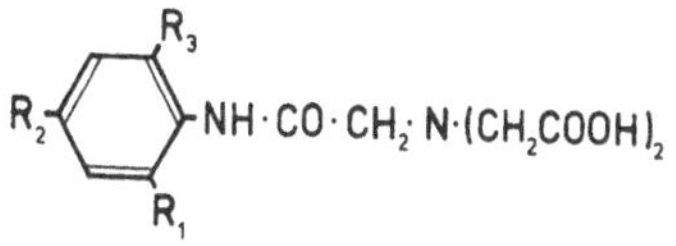

N. acetanilido-iminodiacetic acid

Derivative	R_1	R_2	R_3
Dimethyl-ida	CH_3	H	CH_3
Trimethyl-ida	CH_3	CH_3	CH_3
Diethyl-ida	C_2H_5	H	C_2H_5
p-isopropyl	H	C_3H_7	H
Diisopropyl-ida	C_3H_7	H	C_3H_7
p-n-butyl-ida	C_4H_9	H	H

Fig. 3. N. acetanilido-iminodiacetic acid and its substituents most commonly evaluated as hepato biliary reagents.

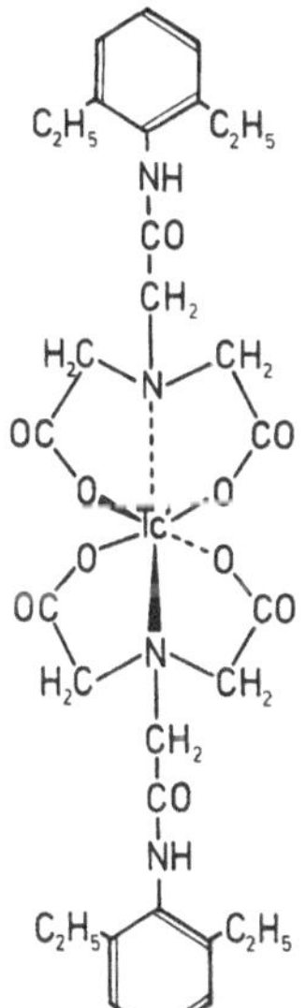

Fig. 4. The most likely structural formula of Diethyl-ida.

36

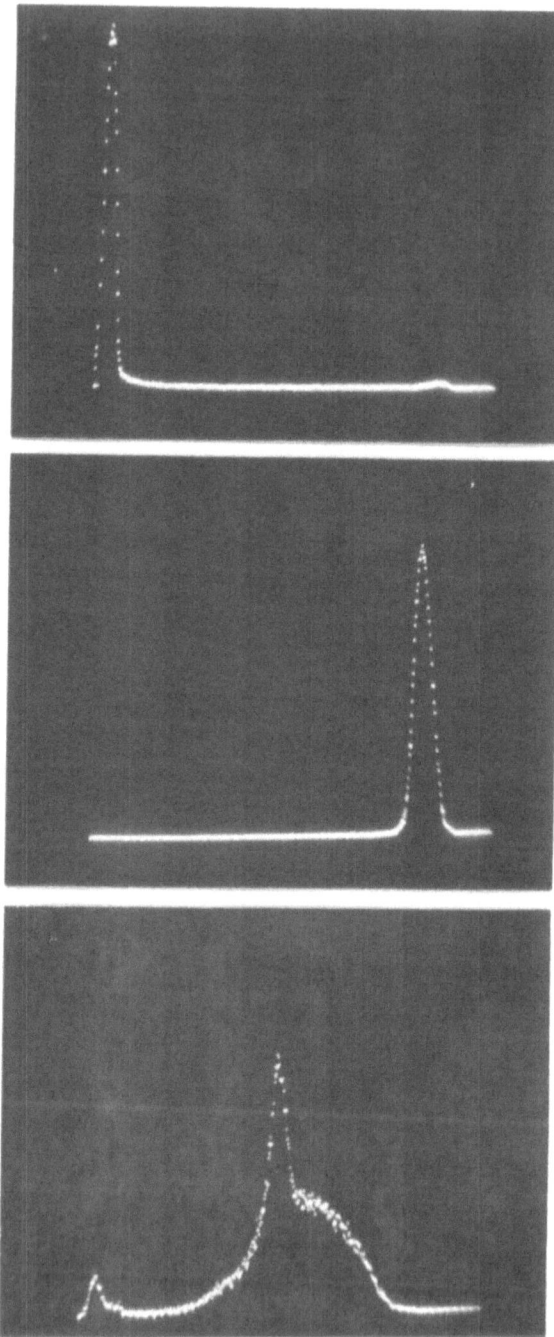

Fig. 5. Profile scans of top: ^{99m}Tc colloid, middle: pertechnetate and lower: ^{99m}Tc-Diethylida (note small amount of colloid and the double Ida peak).

REFERENCES

1. Wistow BW et al, In evaluation of ^{99m}Tc labelled hepatobiliary agents. J. nucl. Med. 18:455, 1977.

2. Loberg MD et al, Development of new radiopharmaceuticals based on N-substitution of Iminodiacetic acid. J. nucl. Med. 17:633, 1976.

3. Subramanian G, Personal communication, 1978.

4. Tjen HSLM, Cholescintigraphy Ph.D. Thesis, University of Utrecht, The Netherlands (in English), 1979.

5. Stöffler G et al, Abdominelle Radioaktivität, Blutspiegel und Kumulative Harnausscheidung vom ^{99m}Tc-di-aethyl-ida (Sn) nach duodenaler Verabreichung. NucComp. 9:70, 1978.

6. Fonda V, Pedersen B, Tc-diethyl-Hida, a contribution to the study of its structure. Eur. J. Nucl. Med. 3:87, 1978.

7. Cox PH, Tjen HSLM, Unpublished data, 1978.

8. Fritzberg AR, Lewis D, HPLC analysis of Tc^{99m} iminodiacetate Hepatobiliary agents and a question of multiple peaks. J. nucl. Med. 21:1180, 1980.

9. Loberg MD, Fields AT, Chemical structure of technetium 99m labelled N-(2-6-dimethylphenylcarbamoylmethyl)imunodiacetic acid. Int. J. appl. Radiat. 29:167, 1978.

10. Libson K, Deutsch E, Barnett BL, Structural characterisation of a ^{99m}Tc diphosphonate complex. J. Amer. Chem. Soc. 102:7:2476, 1980.

11. De Kieviet W, Recent Developments in Technetium chemistry. Identification of the structure of various complexes and relation to biological activity. Nucl. Med. XX 1:2, 1981.

12. Cox PH, Solid Phase Labelling - An improved method for the preparation of Technetium labelled Radiopharmaceuticals. Proceedings IAEA symposium Medical Radio Nuclide Imaging, Heidelberg, 1980. In print.

13. Cox PH, Recent Developments in Technetium Kits. Nucl. Med. XX 1:6, 1981.

14. Frier M, Hesslewood SR, Quality Assurance of Radiopharmaceuticals, London, Chapman and Hall, 1980.

15. Solco-Hida. Product information book, Solco Nuclear Basle, 1979.

16. Parson RBR, Cel Chromatography scanning, a method for the identification and quality control of technetium radiopharmaceuticals. Report Luri 01, 1974.

17. Heide L, Stamm A, Bögl W, Analytik radiochemische Verunreinigungen in Radiopharmaka. Teil II. STH Berichte, Berlin, Dietrich Reimer Verlag, p 92, 1980.

18. Fritzberg AR, Huckaby D, Development and Results routine quality control procedures for Tc^{99m}-Iminodiacetic hepatobiliary agents. 1980. In print.

19. Fritzberg AR, Lewis D, HPLC analysis of Tc^{99m} iminodiacetic hepatobiliary agents and a question of multiple peaks. J. nucl. Med. 21:1180, 1980.

20. Zivanovic MA et al, The stability and distribution of Tc-Hida in vivo and in vitro. Eur. J. Nucl. Med. 9:369, 1979.

21. De Schrijver M, Personal communication, 1978.

4. THE RADIOPHARMACOLOGICAL BEHAVIOUR OF IDA-DERIVATIVES IN NORMAL EXPERIMENTAL ANIMALS

P.H. COX

4.1. INTRODUCTION

Whilst Technetium-Ida derivatives all show basically similar patterns of biodistribution and as such are suited for cholescintigraphy they nevertheless differ significantly enough from each other to have warranted more detailed comparisons to select the reagent most suited for cholescintigraphy in humans.

A review of the basic biological behaviour in animals immediately demonstrates that not only are there observable differences between derivatives but there are also differences in the biological behaviour of any one derivative in different species of animal. Animal data does not therefore directly relate to human biodistribution although many qualitative resemblances can be found.

4.2. Biodistribution in animals blood clearance and liver uptake

Following intravenous injection all Ida-derivatives are rapidly removed from the blood stream by the hepatocytes. A small percentage is cleared by the kidneys. The amount excreted in the urine varies but does not appear to be related to the rate of blood clearance, p-butyl-Ida for example has a much slower blood clearance than Diethyl-Ida but is excreted to a lower extent in the urine. After entering the hepatocytes the reagents are rapidly excreted into the bile and pass to the intestine and gall-bladder. When comparing transport rates from the hepatocytes to the intestine it should be borne in mind, with respect to rat data, that the rat has no gall-bladder.

Loberg (1) demonstrated in mice and dogs that approximately 80 - 87% of Tc^{99m}-Dimethyl-Ida entered the hepatocytes. The blood clearance was rapid, in mice only 3% of the injected dose remained in the blood stream 5 minutes post injection and less than 1% at 30 minutes. The blood clearance in the dog was much slower 3% being present at 30 minutes post injection. Similar results were reported by Ryan (2) and Chiotellis (3). Wistow (4) compared several Ida-derivatives with ^{131}I-Rose Bengal and Tc[99m]-Pyridoxal complexes in the baboon. Once again the results differed from those observed in mice and dogs. Tc[99m]-Diethyl-Ida showed the most rapid blood clearance and the highest biliary concentration 30 minutes post injection, 4 times that of Rose Bengal and almost twice that of Dimethyl-Ida. The total amounts of Dimethyl- and Diethyl-Ida excreted in the bile were almost identical indicating that the discrepancy is relative to the rate of blood clearance.

Chiotellis (3) compared Tc[99m]-Dimethyl-Ida with ^{131}I-Rose Bengal and concluded that although blood clearance rates were similar the rate of accumulation of the Ida-derivative in the gall-bladder was more rapid. Smith (5) examined the kinetics of Tc[99m]-Dimethyl-Ida, Tc[99m]-Pyridoxylene glutamate and ^{131}I-Rose Bengal in the rat and reported that the blood disappearance was a three exponential curve for the first two reagents (representing liver, tissue and urine extraction) and two for Rose Bengal.

4.3. Renal clearance

The urinary clearance of Ida-derivatives is comparatively small and does not interfere with clinical studies, indeed the appearance of renal activity on Diethyl-Ida scintigrams can be used as a diagnostic sign of decreased blood clearance. Subramanian (6) investigated the effect of structural formula changes on the biodistribution in rabbits and demonstrated that these influence renal clearance ratio the more lipophilic the molecule the smaller the renal clearance. Zivanovic(7) observed sex linked differences in the renal clearance rates of Tc[99m]-Dimethyl-Ida in rats and suggested that this may be hormonal linked.

4.4. The mechanism of hepatocyte clearance

As has been pointed out in chapter 3 whilst derivatives of Ida have structures analogous to that of lidocaine it is clear that they follow a different metabolic pathway.

Loberg (1) suggested that the hepatobiliary clearance of Dimethyl-Ida was due to an affinity of the hepatocytes for lipophylic chelating groups. Subramanian (6) confirmed that the liver uptake could be influenced by altering the structural formula. Increasing the lipophilicity of the molecule increased biliary excretion and reduced urinary excretion. Progressive substitution of the Methyl 2 - 6 groups to Isopropyl increased hepatocyte concentration of the reagent but decreased biliary excretion.

Cox (8) demonstrated that the maximum time of uptake in the rat liver and T½ for the excretory phase could be related to the molecular weight of the complexes and also suggested that p- substituted molecules showed slower turn-over rates than other derivatives of similar molecular weight. Diethyl-Ida showed the most rapid liver uptake and bile excretion, p-butyl the slowest, confirming observations in humans. The smaller the molecule the more rapid the turnover. A further possibility is that the charge on the molecule will also influence hepatocyte uptake (9).

Chiotellis (10) investigated N-substituted carbamoyl iminodiacetates and their biological distribution in mice. It was concluded that the biodistribution was affected by structure, polarity and molecular weight. Liver affinity appeared to decrease as the polarity of the molecule increased, substitution in the o-position increased urinary elimination and alkoxy or isometric alkyl substitution speeded up the in vivo kinetics.

4.5. Intra hepatic metabolism

As has already been mentioned lidocaine is metabolized in the liver to monoethylglycine and xylidine of which the latter is excreted via the kidneys and the former in the bile; reabsorption may occur from the intestines. This is clearly not the case with Diethyl-Ida and other Ida-derivatives.

Zivanovic (7) demonstrated that the small amounts of Dimethyl-Ida excreted in the urine was unchanged. Loberg (1) reinjected Dimethyl-Ida extracted from the urine and gall-bladder and concluded from the fact that the biodistribution patterns were the same as the original compound that it passed through the liver and kidneys unchanged. Tjen (11) however observed that Diethyl-Ida complexes readily with bile salts and therefore it would not be possible to determine whether this occurs in the hepatocyte or in the bile.

The influence of bilirubin on the liver turnover of Ida-derivatives is of some interest. Harvey (12) evaluated the influence of anionic sodium sulpho-bromophthalein and cationic oxyphenonium on the liver turnover of Dimethyl-Ida. It was concluded that Dimethyl-Ida followed a carrier mediated anion pathway and would therefore be susceptible to bilirubin concentrations. Kitani (13,14) confirmed an effect of sulphobromophthalein on Dimethyl-Ida turnover. Porter et al (15) used isolated hepatocytes to study the uptake of hepatobiliary agents and confirmed that raised bilirubin concentration levels depressed the uptake of Ida-derivatives.

Fritzberg (16) also carried out studies analogous to those of Harvey with similar results.

4.6. Intestinal reabsorption

No measurable intestinal reabsorption has been reported. To study this we introduced Pertechnetate into the duodenum of anaesthatized rats as control and Diethyl-Ida into the duodenum of another group. One hour post injection the animals were sacrificed and the liver and blood concentrations were determined. The Pertechnetate group showed blood levels of 0.14% dose (m) and liver concentrations of 0.32% dose/mg the figures for Diethyl-Ida were 0.01% per ml blood and 0.01% mg liver.

The study was repeated using the intestinal activity from a rat previously injected intravenously with Diethyl-Ida. The intestinal contents were introduced into the duodenum of a second rat. One hour later no significant blood or liver activity could be measured.

4.7. Conclusions

Although animal studies show considerable interspecies variation in the biological behaviour of Ida-derivatives there is a qualiatative relationship which enables some conclusions to be drawn which are relevant to man.

Technetium labeled Ida-derivatives are preferentially incorporated into hepatocytes after intravenous injection and are rapidly excreted into the bile. There is a limited urinary excretion which is related to the polarity of the complex. Increasing polarity is reflected in reduced urinary excretion increased liver concentration but reduced bile clearance rates. The rate of uptake in the hepatocyte decreases with increasing molecular weight as does the rate of excretion into the bile. The lower molecular weight complexes such as Diethyl-Ida and p-isopropyl-Ida show the most rapid liver uptake and clearance into bile and therefore would appear to be the reagents of choice for clinical studies.

These compounds are not reabsorbed after excretion into the intestines. Many authors consider them to be excreted unchanged but there is evidence that they are bound to bile salts.

The higher molecular weight compounds such as p-butyl-Ida are poorly excreted via the kidneys even when delayed blood clearance is present whereas Diethyl and p-isopropyl-Ida show increased urinary excretion under such circumstances. For this reason it has been suggested that in severely jaundiced patients a better visualization of liver parenchyma may be obtained by using p-butyl-Ida. The liver does indeed show better contrast with the back-ground under these conditions but the turnover rates are too slow for good evaluation of changes in liver function in follow-up studies. All Ida-derivatives appear to follow an anionic metabolic pathway and are influenced by bilirubin levels.

REFERENCES

1. Loberg MD et al, Development of new radiopharmaceuticals based on N-substitution of iminodiacetic acid. J. nucl. Med. 17:633, 1976.

2. Ryan J et al, Technetium-99m-labelled N (216-dimethylcarbamoyl methyl) iminodiacetic acid: A new radiopharmaceutical for hepatobiliary imaging studies.
   J. nucl. Med. 17:545, 1977.

3. Chiotellis E et al, 99^mTc-Hida a gall-bladder imaging agent. Experimental
   aspects. Eur. J. nucl. Med. 3:41, 1978.

4. Wistow BW et al, An evaluation of 99^mTc-hepatobiliary imaging agents. J. nucl.
   Med. 18:455, 1977.

5. Smith RB et al, Pharmacokinetics of hepatobiliary imaging agents in rats.
   J. nucl. Med. 20:45, 1979.

6. Subramanian G et al, The influence of structural changes on biodistribution
   of 99^mTc N-substituted Ida derivatives. In: Nuklearmedizin. Proceedings
   15th International Congress Society of Nuclear Medicine (Europe). Schmidt
   HAE, Woldring MG (eds), Groningen, 1977.

7. Zivanovic M et al, The stability and distribution of Tc-Hida in vivo and in
   vitro. Eur. J. nucl. Med. 4:369, 1979.

8. Cox PH, The comparative pharmacology of technetium ida derivatives. In:
   Progress in Radiopharmacology. Vol.I. Cox PH (ed), Amsterdam, Elsevier/
   North-Holland Biomedical Press, 1979.

9. Burns D et al, Relationship between molecular structure and biliary excretion
   of Tc99m Hida and Hida analogues. J. nucl. Med. 18:624, 1977.

10. Chiotellis E, Varvarigou A, 99^mTc labelled N-substituted carbamoyl imino-
    diacetates: Relationship between structure and distribution. Int. J. nucl.
    Med. Biol. 7:1, 1980.

11. Tjen HSLM, Cholescintigraphy. Ph.D. Thesis, University of Utrecht, The
    Netherlands (in English), 1979.

12. Harvey E et al, Hepatic clearance mechanism of Tc99m Hida and its effect on
    quantitation of hepato biliary function: consise communication. J. nucl.
    Med. 20:310, 1979.

13. Kitani K et al, Inhibiting effect of sulphobromophthalein (BSP) on the
    hepatic uptake and biliary excretion of 99mTc Hida in rats. Jap. J. nucl.
    Med. 15:999, 1978.

14. Kitani K et al, Inhibiting effect of sulphobromophthalein on the hepatic
    uptake and biliary excretion of 99^mTc-N (2.6 dimethylphenylcarbamoylmethyl)
    diacetic acid and pyridoxylene isoluceine in rats. J. nucl. Med. 20:642,
    1979.

15. Porter DW et al, Comparison of hepatobiliary radiopharmaceuticals in an in
    vitro model. J. nucl. Med. 20:642, 1979.

16. Fritzberg AR et al, Hepatobiliary mechanism of Tc99m-N (2.6 diethylacetani-
    lido)iminodiacarboxylic acid (Diethylida). J. nucl. Med. 20:642, 1979.

5.   RADIOPHARMACOLOGY OF IDA-DERIVATIVES IN EXPERIMENTAL LIVER PARENCHYMAL
     DAMAGE AS WELL AS OBSTRUCTED BILE-DUCTS

H.J. BIERSACK

5.1. INTRODUCTION

Once the significance of cholescintigraphy with Ida-derivatives has been
documented in a large number of publications, mostly from European sources,
a discussion arose concerning the differential diagnosis of parenchymal and
obstructive jaundice. A further question requiring clarification was the
identification of the optimal Ida-derivative. In this respect several groups of
investigators (1,5) performed animal experiments to check on the relevance of
hepatobiliary functional scintigraphy in clearly defined and morphologically
controlable disease patterns such as liver parenchymal damage and obstructive
jaundice.

5.2. Experimental obstructive jaundice

Bähre et al (1) ligated the common bile-duct of 14 mongrel dogs distally
from the junction with the cystic-duct. Pre-operatively as well as immediately
after operation, hepatobiliary functional scintigraphy using Tc^{99m}-Diethyl-Ida
was performed. The duration of the study was up to 3 hours. During a maximum of
7 weeks after ligature, the investigation was repeated weekly. The evaluation
was made on the basis of time-activity curves from the left liver lobe, the left
kidney and a back-ground area (heart region). The time-activity curves over the
liver permitted the determination of the time of maximum accumulation (T max)
and the half-time of excretion ($T\frac{1}{2}$). The interpretation of liver parenchymal
accumulation was done on the basis of the ratio between liver and back-ground
activities (L/B-quotient at T max). In addition, scintigrams permitted the
visual interpretation of activity distribution in liver and bile-ducts. It was
also possible to determine the times of appearance of the radiopharmaceutical
in the liver parenchyma, gall-bladder, kidney and intestine whenever applicable.
The weighing of liver function and the extent of cholestasis were determined
using gamma-GT and GPT, bilirubin and alkaline phosphatase measurements prior to
each cholescintigraphy. In a few cases, 5 weeks after ligature a percutaneous

transhepatic cholangiography and liver histology studies were performed.

5.3. Pre-operative findings (fig. 1)

In all cases prior to the ligature of the common bile-duct, the liver parenchyma was clearly visible 3 to 5 minutes after injection. The T max in the liver was 9 minutes and the half-time of the excretion curve 20 minutes. The gall-bladder was visible approximately 25 minutes after injection. Scintigraphic- ally kidneys could not be observed longer than 15 - 20 minutes after injection. The laboratory values (except for those of bilirubin) were comparable with those found in humans. Bilirubin itself averaging 0.11 mg% was lower than in humans.

5.4. Findings after common bile-duct ligature (fig. 2)

The early postoperative period was characterized by an unmodified visual- ization of the liver in functional scintigraphy. The laboratory values did not change either. The gall-bladder appeared as an extended hot spot and activity passage into the intestine could not be found.

5.5. Findings one to four weeks after ligature (fig. 3)

The excretion half-time was increased to over 30 minutes. The gall-bladder was visible continuously during the entire investigation lasting 3 hours as an accumulation defect in the liver parenchyma. Although there was good accumulation of Ida in the liver parenchyma, no activity appeared in the gall-bladder. In all cases the kidney was scintigraphically visible up to 1 hour after injection. A fifty-fold increase of bilirubin and alkaline phosphatases also indicated a clear-cut cholestasis.

5.6. Findings five to seven weeks after ligature

Five to seven weeks after ligature the gall-bladder continued to be visualized as an accumulation defect in an otherwise well accumulating liver parenchyma. The liver / back-ground ratio which did not change from normal up to 4 weeks after ligature dropped to 2.7 at 5 to 7 weeks after the intervention, i.e. there was a significant increase of liver parenchymal accumulation in comparison to the non-treated dogs. Bilirubin and alkaline phosphatase levels had increased further whereby one has to consider that in the dog a 10 mg% bilirubin level means an increase by a factor 100 of the normal level. Gamma-GT and GPT did not increase to the same extent indicating also in this experimental model a typical cholestasis-enzyme-pattern. Transcutaneous cholangiography (fig.4) 5 weeks after ligature indicated an important enlargement of both intra- and extra-hepatic bile-ducts and a dilated gall-bladder. Histological findings demonstrated canalicular cholestasis and enlarged inflammatory infiltrated periportal areas. The parenchymal uptake of Ida up to 40 days after common bile-duct ligature was still good notwithstanding radiological and laboratory evidence of a significant cholestasis.

This suggests the conclusion that complete obstruction in the dog does not impair accumulation of Diethyl-ida in the liver cell. The criteria for extra-hepatic jaundice in the dog are therefore the absence of activity passage in the gut accompanied by good parenchymal accumulation. In the acute phase, a few hours after extra-hepatic bile-duct obstruction, the gall-bladder is still visualized. In a one-week-old extra-hepatic cholestasis the gall-bladder appears as a filling defect against the parenchyma. In this experimental model, even 7 weeks after ligature, a parenchymal accumulation defect which is found frequently in patients, could not be reproduced.

5.7. Experimental liver parenchymal damage

The same group of investigators (2,3) created hepatic parenchymal damage by a daily injection of 400 mg/kg body weight of Galactosamine in 16 mongrel dogs. Prior to and every second day after the treatment hepatobiliary functional scintigraphy was performed. In addition, scintigrams were made up to a maximum of 3 hours after injection. If 3 hours after injection clear evidence of intestinal passage could not be found, delayed images up to 24 hours after injection were made. Before every functional scintigraphy, serum samples were taken for the determination of bilirubin, alkaline phosphatase, GPT and GOT. The quantitative evaluation was again made using T max and the half-time of the excretion phase as well as the activity ratios of liver and back-ground. In the early phase of the investigation the findings corresponded to those obtained prior to ligature of the common bile-duct: activity was found in the duodenum 40 minutes after injection and in the intestine about 60 minutes after injection.

5.8. Findings after two to four days of Galactosamine treatment

During the first 4 days delays in T max and excretion half-time were found, as well as delayed visualisation of bile-ducts and intestinal tract. The kidneys remained visible for over 45 minutes after injection. Alkaline phosphatase, gamma-GT and bilirubin showed a slight, GPT a more pronounced, increase.

5.9. Findings five to nine days under Galactosamine treatment (fig. 5)

In parallel to the importance of changes of liver histology, the time-activity curves of the liver showed a clear-cut prolongation of T max and T½. Notwithstanding the good visualization of the liver parenchyma, the gall-bladder was not visible in any animal of this group. In addition, a significantly delayed Diethyl-Ida excretion in the gut could be demonstrated in all test-animals. In most cases intestinal excretion could be found only in the late scintigrams. The liver / back-ground ratio decreased significantly to 2.5, the bilirubin increased to approximately 5 mg%. Serum-GPT and GOT increased by factors of 300 and 100 respectively. Notwithstanding this important liver parenchymal damage, Ida-accumulation in the liver was not impaired.

The important finding made in this investigation is that even important liver parenchymal damage does not impair accumulation of Diethyl-Ida, hence in principle in these cases a differential diagnosis of obstructive versus paren-chymal jaundice is possible by checking activity passage into the intestine.

Erjavec et al (4) used carbon tetrachloride to create damage of the hepatic parenchyma. In this study, 1 day after intoxication Ida-accumulation and ex-cretion decreased significantly in agreement with the observed liver damage. A trend to normalization could be observed during consecutive days. In this in-vestigation activity accumulation in the intestine could also be found notwith-standing liver damage.

5.10. Kinetics of different Ida-derivatives in experimental liver damage

Although different animal species possess different biliary elimination patterns for organic anions (5), it has been demonstrated that the kinetics of biliary excretion is simular in humans, monkeys and rabbits (6), hence exper-imental animal data yields conclusions which can be transposed to the human being. Popescu et al (5) also used carbon tetrachloride to create liver paren-chymal damage just as Erjavec et al (4) but in the rabbit. Different Tc^{99m}-labeled Ida-derivatives were tested in this animal model in order to investigate which derivative possessed the most pronounced accumulation and excretion in the prescence of liver cell damage. The oral application of carbon tetrachloride was made 17 to 18 hours prior to the investigation. Shortly before the injection of the radiopharmaceutical, the hepatic-duct was canulated in order to collect liver bile continuously. In addition, bilirubin, aldolase and transaminase levels were determined. The liver findings were documented histologically.

Different Ida-derivatives were tested using this model and their kinetics compared: Dimethyl-, Diethyl-, p-isopropyl-, Trimethyl-, Diisopropyl- and p-n-butyl-Ida. It was demonstrated that experimental liver cell damage reduced biliary elimination with all Ida-derivatives. Trimethyl-Ida had the best kinetics in untreated controls, but in the CCl_4-treated animals its excretion dropped significantly. In contrast, Diethyl-Ida was found to have the highest accumulative biliary excretion in the prescence of parenchymal damage. Comparable results were found only using Diisopropyl-Ida. The results of Popescu et al (5) therefore suggest the superiority of Diethyl-Ida as hepatobiliary radiopharmaceutical.

The investigations performed by different groups permit the conclusion that the differences in kinetics of Ida-derivatives allow differential diagnosis regarding the etiology of jaundice. Especially, the results in liver parenchymal damage show that notwithstanding important hepatocellular changes with significantly increased transaminase and bilirubin levels, excretion into the intestine can be found, because usually there are still a few hepatocytes present which are still able to accumulate and excrete Ida-derivatives. This excretion then leads to a scintigraphically detectable radioactivity accumulation in the intestine. Hence a differential diagnosis is possible, even in the prescence of massively increased bilirubin levels, when delayed images are made up to 24 hours after injection.

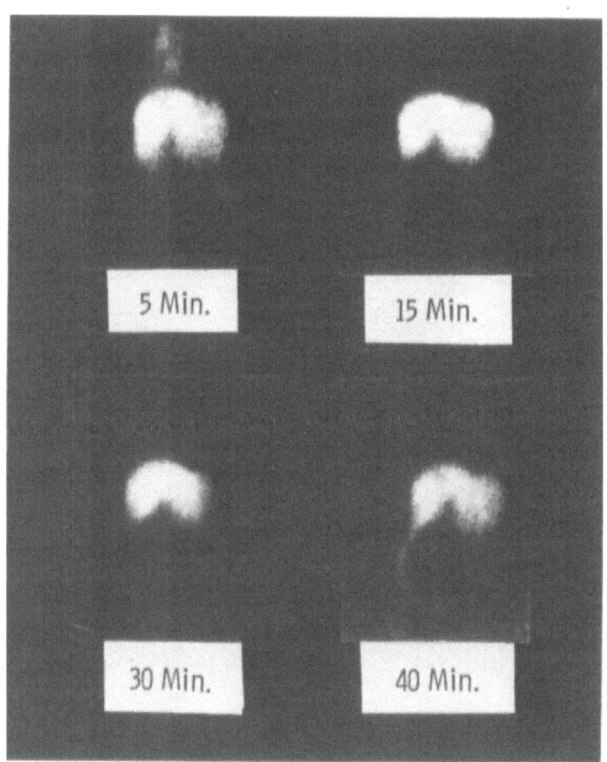

Fig. 1. Scintigraphy with Tc^{99m}-Ida in a normal dog.

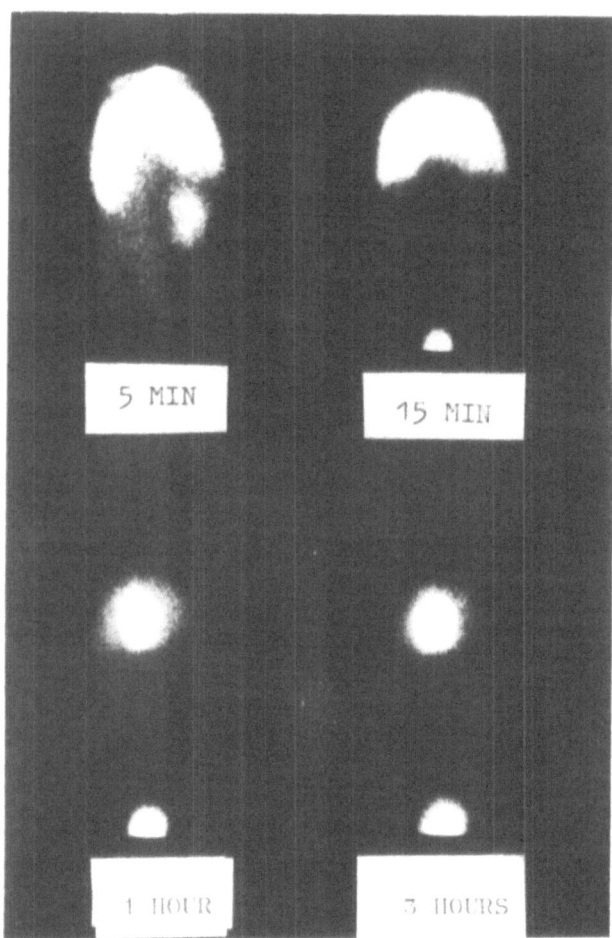

Fig. 2. Scintigraphy with Tc^{99m}-Ida immediately after ligature of the common bile duct: no bile discharge into the intestines, gall-bladder appears as a "hot spot".

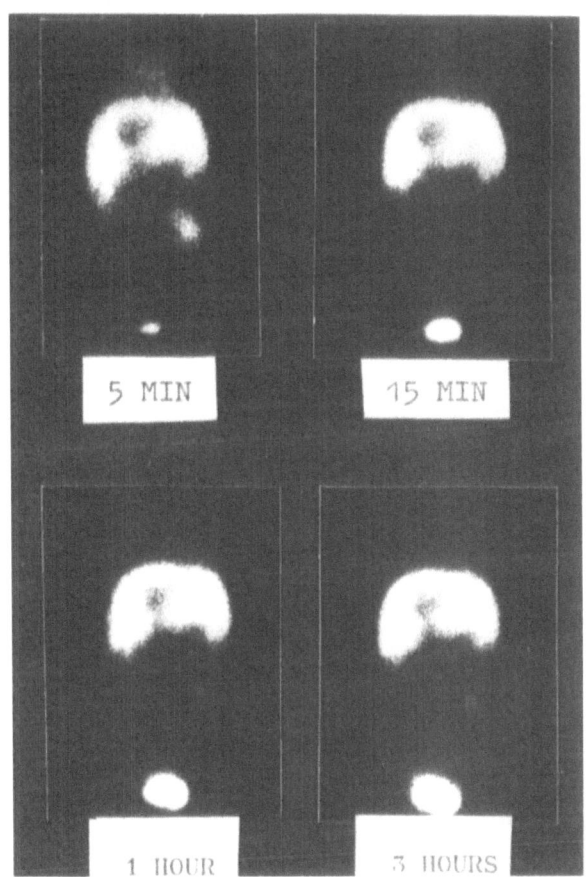

Fig. 3. Scintigraphy with Tc^{99m}-Ida 1 to 4 weeks after ligature of the common bile duct: no bile discharge into the intestines, gall-bladder appears as a "cold spot".

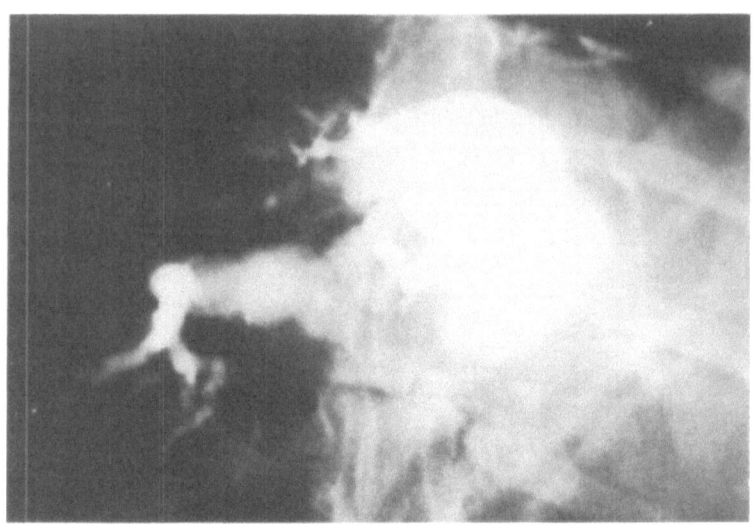

Fig. 4. PTC 5 weeks after ligature of the common bile duct: dilated bile ducts and gall-bladder.

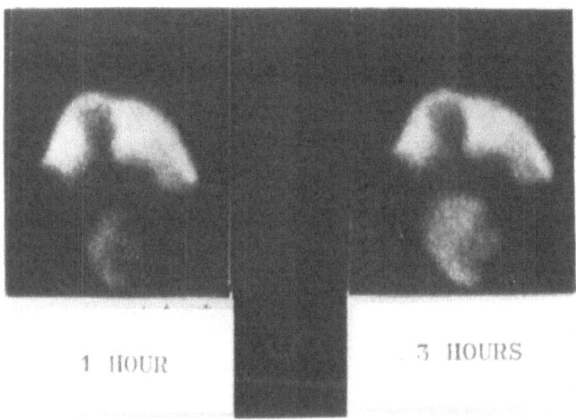

Fig. 5. Scintigraphy with Tc^{99m}-Ida 5 to 9 days under Galactosamine treatment: regular discharge of the bile into the intestines, no accumulation of the tracer in the gall-bladder.

REFERENCES

1. Bähre M, Biersack HJ, Breuel HP, Tierexperimentelle Untersuchungen mit ^{99m}Tc-Diäthyl-Hida bei akutem komplettem Gallengangsverschluss. Nucl. Med. 18:215, 1979.

2. Bähre M, Biersack HJ, Breuel HP, Tierexperimentelle Untersuchungen mit ^{99m}Tc-Diäthyl-Hida bei Galaktosamin-Hepatitis. In: Nuklearmedizin, die klinische Relevanz der Nuklearmedizin. Schmidt HAE, Riccabona G (eds), Stuttgart, New York, Schattauer.

3. Bähre M, Biersack HJ, Hofmann S, Cholescintigraphy in experimentally induced obstructive and parenchymatous jaundice. In: Progress in Radiopharmacology, Vol. I. Cox PH (ed), Amsterdam, Elsevier/North-Holland Biomedical Press, 1979.

4. Erjavec M, Pahor S, Simcic V, Computer assisted clearance calculations of diethyl-Ida in dogs induced liver damage. In: Progress in Radiopharmacology, Vol I. Cox PH (ed), Amsterdam, Elsevier/North-Holland Biomedical Press, 1979.

5. Popescu HI, Chia HL, Peter F, Biliary elimination of various N-(acetanilido)-iminodiacetic acid (Ida) derivatives in rabbits with induced liver cell damage. In: Progress in Radiopharmacology, Vol. I. Cox PH (ed), Amsterdam, Elsevier/North-Holland Biomedical Press, 1979.

6. Smith RL, The excretory function of bile. Chapman and Hall, London, p.14.

6. THE BIOKINETICS OF Tc^{99m} LABELED HEPATOBILIARY AGENTS IN HUMANS

G.F. Fueger

6.1. INTRODUCTION

Hepatobiliary agents with Tc^{99m} are tracers of bile flow, of bile storage in the gall bladder, of hepatocyte metabolism, of gastrointestinal propagation or of reflux from duodenum (or ileum) into the stomach; the latter objectives require rapid arrival of a sufficient amount of tracer in the duodenum (fig.1). A relatively large number of Tc^{99m} labeled hepatobiliary tracers have been described in the scientific literature:

Derivatives of N- (Phenylcarbamoylmethyl) iminodiacetic acid (1,2)

Dihydro-thioctic acid (DHT) (3)

Mercaptoisobutyric acid (4)

Pyridoxylidene Glutamate (PyG) (5)

Pyridoxal Leucine (OyL) (5,6,7,8)

Pyridoxalphenylalanin (9,10)

8-Hydroxy-quinolin-7-carboxylate (11)

D-Penicillamine (12)

Tetracycline (13)

Toluidine blue (14)

The list of Tc^{99m} agents which are predominately eliminated from the body via the hepatobiliary route, is likely to grow, since excretion via liver and bile is the normal excretory pathway for lipidsoluble compounds and organic anions with a molecular weight greater than approximately 300, due to the fact that the kidney cannot handle such compounds efficiently. Many such substances, however, undergo elimination via bile *and* urine. The development of derivatives of N-(Phenylcarbamoylmethyl) iminodiacetic acid was initiated by Loberg's (15) introduction of the bifunctional chelate 2,6-Dimethylacetanilidoiminodiacetic acid. "Bifunctional", since the chelate fulfills two functions: 1. the 2,6-Dimethylacetanilido part of the molecule promotes uptake into the liver (hepatotropism) and excretion into bile (cholaffinity) and 2. the iminodiacetate part

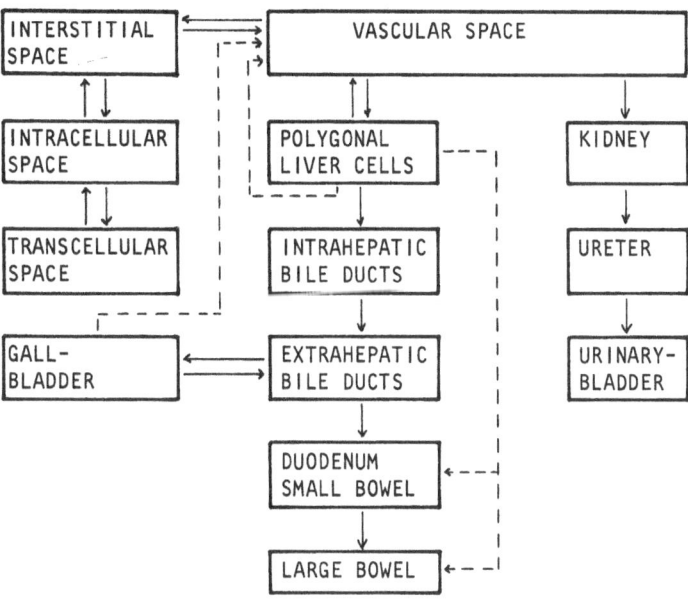

Fig. 1. Hepato biliary tracers. Pathways and spaces.

of the molecule facilitates the chelation of some cationic species of reduced Tc^{99m}. The term Hepatoiminiodiacetate was shortened to HIDA

The two methyl groups of the N-substituted acetanilidoiminodiacetate were exchanged for other groups very quickly: substitution was made on one or more carbon atoms of the benzene ring, position 1 being the point of attachment to the rest of the molecule and the name was changed to N-"X"-phenylcarbomoyl-methyl)-iminodiacetate to confirm with the systematic chemical nomenclature. The following derivatives have been evaluated and used for clinical investiga-tions. (The part of the name in italics corresponds to "X"):

N-(2,6-*dimethyl*-phenylcarbamoylmethyl)-Ida   Loberg's HIDA (15)

N-(2,4,6-*trimethyl*-phenylcarbamoylmethyl)-Ida   TRIMIDA (HOECHST)

N-(2,6-*diethyl*-phenylcarbamoylmethyl-Ida   HEPATOBIDA, SOLCO-HIDA; BIDA
                                       (German-authors), DIAIDA, DE-IDA
                                       EHIDA

N-(2,6-*diisopropyl*-phenylcarbamoylmethyl-Ida   DISIDA

N-(4-*isopropyl*-phenylcarbamoylmethyl-Ida   PIPIDA,p-isopropyl

N-(4-n-*butyl*-phenylcarbamoylmethyl)-Ida   BIDA (US and Canadian authors)
"p-butyl"

The compounds will be referred to below only by the "X" part of their name which is given in italics above.

The biological behaviour of these compounds can be evaluated from several points of view, such as accuracy in the elucidation of a special dysfunction, usefulness for the measurement of liver blood flow, or total liver function, shortest possible time interval to complete a study, demonstration of bile flow and its impairment, identification of focal regions with impaired function, or the estimation of cumulative activities, i.e. fractions of administered radio-actives and residence times in focal regions with significantly altered function.

6.2. The principle pattern of biological distribution

The new Tc^{99m} hepatobiliary reagents, particularly the so called HIDA or IDA derivatives, already undergo hepatic uptake while the initial dilution after intravenous injection is still taking place. Exposure to the hepatocytes which extract these tracers with evident high extraction efficiencies depends upon liver blood flow through the hepatic artery and portal vein. Accumulation within hepatic parenchyma will be the result of and proportional to liver blood flow, extraction efficiency and number of functioning hepatocytes. Hepatocytes contain storage proteins, Y and Z; they also have the metabolic ability to

render lipids watersoluble by conjugation. Different hepatobiliary tracers can
be expected to pass the hepatocytes at different rates since they may be bound
to various degrees to the intracellular storage proteins or may require conjugation prior to their secretion via the biliary pole of the hepatocyte into the
biliary canaliculus. The creation of bile is a continuous process which can be
increased to some extent by choleretics, such as bile acids. The hepatobiliary
tracers mix with bile in the canaliculus, and are transported into the main bile
ducts, into the gall-bladder and duodenum together with the bile and its other
constituents.

Congenital deficiencies of hepatocytic uptake at the parenchymal pole,
deficiency of conjugation, and deficiency in secretion can be expected to
influence the elimination of some hepatobiliary reagents. There are more open
questions than answers. From the clinical observation of conjugated hyperbilirubinemia it must be expected that hepatobiliary reagents may be returned into
the blood stream after having been taken up by hepatocytes. This return may
take place either directly of indirectly via the biliary pole and canaliculus.

Biliary obstruction with its accompanying increase in intraductal pressure
halts biliary secretion at pressures above 35 ml H_2O, and the elimination of
hepatobiliary reagents will similarly cease. Hepatitis, toxic hepatopathies and
steatosis can be associated with jaundice indicative of an impaired elimination
of bilirubin. Hepatobiliary reagents can be expected to be retained as well.
Under such conditions; they can further be expected to undergo a delayed
elimination from the hepatocytes before jaundice develops if they are sensitive
indicators of the eliminatory hepatic metabolism. The latter is regarded as the
most sensitive of all liver-functions and therefore the demonstration of its
impairment is the most reliable early sign of hepatic parenchymal dysfunction.
As long as the secretion of bile is maintained, and as long as hepatobiliary
reagents follow bile in sufficiently high concentration to enable imaging, these
compounds will demonstrate impairment of bile flow and bile storage in the gall-
bladder.

If there is impairment of hepatic uptake or biliary secretion there may
diminished hepatic reagent uptake from the blood or increased return to the
blood stream so that relatively higher blood levels prevail for longer periods
of time. The kidneys probably eliminate hepatobiliary reagents with specific
extraction efficiencies, and even if the renal extraction fraction is small the
persistence of relatively high or higher than normal blood levels will result in
seemingly increased urinary elimination of a hepatobiliary reagent.

The gall-bladder possesses the ability to concentrate bile by reabsorption of water and salt. Will hepatobiliary reagents also be reabsorbed? Probably yes. There is the enterohepatic recirculation of bile acids. Will the hepatobiliary agents join this pathway? Probably no, since it was shown not to be the case with Diethylida. The principle question is do the new Tc^{99m} labeled hepato-biliary reagents behave alike or not, and if they do, to what degree do they differ from each other? As this review will show there are more open questions than answers.

The physiological spaces and the processes involved in the biological distribution of hepatobiliary radiotracers are listed below:

Principle pattern of biological distribution of hepatobiliary radiotracers:	
Compartment:	Process:
Intravascular space	Dilution after injection
Extracellular space	Diffusion (to and fro)
Hepatocytes	Extraction from blood
Hepatocytes	Transfer, storage
Hepatocytes	Secretion
Hepatocytes	Return into vascular space
Bile ducts	Drainage
Biliary canaliculi	Reflux into vascular space
Gall-bladder	Storage
Gall-bladder	Reabsorption into vascular space
Intestinal tract	Propagation
Intestinal tract	Reabsorption into vascular space
Renal parenchyma	Filtration, secretion?
Urinary tract	Drainage

6.3. Blood

Total blood volume: The sum of the volumes of the various types of circulating blood cells and plasma is cells: 46% by volume, plasma 54% by volume. Total volume (ml) in adults: $85.27 \times W$ (kg) $- 25$, where W is body weight.
Reference adult:

Total blood volume: male 5200 ml, female 3900 ml
Weight of total blood: male 5500 g, female 4100 g
ICRP 1975 (16).

Principle reagent behaviour: After a single intravenous injection there is the customary precipitous fall in concentration followed by a slow continous disappearance which needs at least 3, probably 4 exponential functions to be analyzed if followed to 24 hours post injection.

Parameters evaluated: Arterio-venous concentration difference as % dose in blood. Halftime in blood (sample measurements). Halftimes in blood and inter-stitial space (surface activity measurements). Reagent retention in blood (sample measurements). Reagent retention in blood and interstitial space (surface activity). Distribution volumes. Clearance estimates (distribution volume x k).

Arteriovenous concentration difference: In a patient with cirrhosis the time course of Tc^{99m} Diethyl-Ida was plotted from concentration measurements in plasma samples obtained from catheterization of the femoral artery and hepatic vein, following a simple injection of Diethyl-Ida. The concentration was ex-pressed in counts/sec x ml; the time courses in the arterial and venous samples paralleled each other, the difference was virtually constant. The measurement was carried out to 40 minutes post injection (17). It is a difficult to draw a definitive conclusion about the kinetics of the uptake of Tc^{99m} Diethyl-Ida in the liver. The almost constant uptake rate and the decreasing extraction frac-tion argue strongly against first order kinetics. The kinetics by means of which Tc^{99m} Diethyl-Ida is taken up in the liver is complex in parenchymal disorders. The process seems to deviate from first order kinetics with the usual dose of the reagent.

The hepatic extraction fraction of Tc^{99m} Diethyl-Ida has a wide range in patients with parenchymal disorders of the liver. In the individual patient, the extraction fraction depends on the arterial concentration. In parenchymal liver disease, Tc^{99m} Diethyl-Ida is probably not handled by bilirubin independent processes. The volume of distribution corresponds most likely to the extra-cellular volume.

Halftime in blood: (sample measurements). Normal subjects: Dimethyl, blood-samples (number 12): component I: 4.6 ± 1.0 minutes, component II: 31 ± 7.0 minutes, observation mode to 60 minutes post injection (18). Diethyl, plasma-samples (number 10): component I: (0-3 minutes post injection: 2.64 ± 0.7 minutes, component II: not estimated, component III: (17-30 minutes post injection): 20.67 ± 4.85 minutes, observation to 30 minutes post injection (19).

Percentage dose in blood:

Normal subjects (number = 12), Dimethyl (18)

15	30	45	60 minutes post injection
16	9	7	5 percentage dose in blood

Calculated from graph. Figures from text for blood dose at 5 minutes: 32 ± 4.9%; at 60 minutes; 5.1 ± 2.8%

Normal subjects (number = 6) Diethyl (20)

3	5	7	10	15	45	90	180 minutes post injection
4.5	3.3	2.5	1.9	1.5	0.8	0.5	0.35 percentage dose/l weight

Cirrhotic patients (number = 8) Diethyl and p-isopropyl (22) plasma samples:

time	3	5	10	20	30	45	60 minutes post injection
Diethyl	12.6±2.9	9.5±3.3	7.2±3.0	4.9±2.4	3.4±1.0	1.7±0.8	2.3±0.9 percentage dose/l weight
p-isopropyl	14.7±3.5	11.5±1.95	9.6±1.6	6.7±2.1	5.9±1.9	4.6±1.8	4.3±1.7 "

Normal subjects (number = 4) Diethyl (21)

30'	60'	120'	180'	240' minutes post injection
1.001	0.746	0.508	0.443	0.385 percentage dose/l weight

Cholestatic patients (number = 20) Diethyl and p-butyl (23) plasma samples:

Bilirubin levels: 3.2 - 25 mg/dl alkaline Phosphate levels: 250 - 1230

	3	5	10	15	20	30	60	180 minutes post injection
Diethyl	11.4±4.2	8.8±3.9	7.9±3.3	6.6±3.2	6.3±3.1	5.6±2.7	4.4±2.15	2.4±1.5 percentage dose/l weight
p-butyl	16.1±4.8	13.0±4.25	10.2±3.6	9.0±3.35	8.0±3.0	6.9±2.8	4.85±2.2	3.5±2.0 "

Patients with hepatocellular or obstructive jaundice

Dimethyl (number = 4)
Component I: 5.3 ± 0.7 minutes, component II: 118 ± 36 minutes, observed to 75 minutes post injection (18)

Patients with biliary obstruction average total bilirubin 5 mg%)

Diethyl (number = 10) plasma samples
Component I: (0-3 minutes post injection): 3.0 ± 11.9 minutes, component II: not estimated, component III: (17-30 minutes post injection): 25.6 ± 145 minutes, observed to 30 minutes (19).

Patients with nonobstructive hepatic parenchymal or biliary secretory impairment (average total bilirubin 12 mg%):

Diethyl (number = 34) plasma samples
Component I: (0-3 minutes post injection): 1.1 ± 7.2 minutes, component II: not estimated, component III (17-30 minutes post injection): 12.3 ± 91.4 minutes (19).

Indices of reagent retention in blood or plasma (sample measurements):
Diethyl, calculation of (cpm/ml blood t=20)/(cpm/ml blood t=5)
10 normal subjects   : 0.5 ± 0.05
12 patients with cirrhosis   : 0.55 ± 0.05
 7 patients with extrahepatic obstruction: 0.67 ± 0.05 (24)

Diethyl, calculation of (cpm/ml plasma t=30)/(cpm/ml plasma t=3)
normal subjects (number = 10)   : 0.154 ± 0.002
biliary obstruction (average)
total bilirubin 5 mg/dl (number = 10)   : 0.45 ± 0.117
hepatocellular or biliary
secretory impairment (number = 34)   : 0.222 ± 0.088
(average total bilirubin 12 mg%) (19)

Tracer retention in blood plus interstitial space:
(Measurements of surface activity)

Diethyl, calculation of (counts ROI heart t=20)/(counts ROI heart t=5)

16 normal subjects	: 0.562 ± 0.043 (25)
8 patients with cholelithiasis without obstruction	: 0.59 ± 0.032 (25)
6 patients with cholecystectomy and without calculi	: 0.577 ± 0.050 (25)

Diethyl, calculation of precordial countrate ratio (26)

condition	number	counts at t=3 counts at t max	counts at t=15 counts at t max
normal	50	0.13 ± 0.09	0.085 ± 0.05
steatosis	25	0.21 ± 0.15	0.18 ± 0.13
cirrhosis	25	0.38 ± 0.22	0.26 ± 0.15
complete obstruction	15	0.49 ± 0.42	0.32 ± 0.29
incomplete obstruction	35	0.27 ± 0.18	0.17 ± 0.10
obstruction and cholangitis	18	0.31 ± 0.26	0.23 ± 0.17

The above parameter is an index of tracer retention in blood. The more pronounced the hepatic pathological changes the higher the index. This parameter is not useful for the differentiation of jaundice, but has been recommended for the follow-up of total hepatic function (26)

Calculation of (counts ROI heart t=10)/(counts ROI heart t=2) (27)

	number	Ida-derivatives	ratio
normal subjects	20	Diethyl	0.55 ± 0.10
" "	20	Diisopropyl	0.48 ± 0.11
" "	9	Diisopropyl	0.44 ± 0.07
" "	9	p-butyl	0.55 ± 0.08
hyperbilirubinemia			
1 - 5 mg/dl	16	Diethyl	0.58 ± 0.12
" "	16	Diisopropyl	0.53 ± 0.08
" "	17	Diisopropyl	0.53 ± 0.14
" "	17	p-butyl	0.58 ± 0.14
hyperbilirubinemia			
5 mg/dl	8	Diethyl	0.69 ± 0.07
"	8	Diisopropyl	0.68 ± 0.05
"	8	Diisopropyl	0.59 ± 0.04
"	7	p-butyl	0.76 ± 0.12

Distribution volumes:

Initial fictitious distribution volume: activity injected/(cpm/ml at t=0)

Diethyl (19)

	number	value
normal subjects	10	3344 ± 1088 ml
biliary obstruction (average bilirubin 5 mg/dl)	10	3767 ± 1134 ml
hepatocellular impairment, (average bilirubin 12 mg/dl)	34	4067 ± 1265 ml

17 - 30 minutes fictitious distribution volume:

Diethyl (19)

	number	value
normal subjects	10	18809 ± 7281
biliary obstruction (average bilirubin 5 mg/dl)	10	8472 ± 3222
hepatocellular impairment (average bilirubin 12 mg/dl)	34	14540 ± 6554

6.4. Clearance estimates (distribution volume x k)

Diethyl, 4 mCi intravenously, ROI-heart, ROI-body back-ground (= total
field of vision of scintillation camera less liver and intestinal tracer depots),
225 frames of 12 seconds each, 45 minutes total. Time, activity curves in ROI-
heart and ROI-bgd corrected for decay, calculation of clearance values based on
comparment model using 3 exponential functions between t=0 and 45 minutes post
injection, 45 patients with (a) no hepatic pathology, (b) hepatic parenchymal
dysfunction, (c) parenchymal jaundice, (d) obstructive jaundice: since the time
activity curves in ROI heart and ROI body do not undergo a continous single-
exponential decay very different clearance values are obtained dependent upon
the time interval from which the elimination constant is taken. The clearance
values started high, diminished successively, ran through a shallow minimum
between about 20 and 30 minutes post injection and rose again thereafter. This
general behaviour showed no dependence upon pathology; the actual values, and
the time of the minimum, however, did so.

The authors conclude that the rates of all exchange processes between the
various distribution spaces of Diethyl reach a minimum at about 17 minutes in
normal subjects, at about 25 minutes in hepatic parenchymal dysfunction, at
about 29 minutes in parenchymal jaundice, and at about 33 minutes in obstructive
jaundice (28).

Biological elimination constants from sample measurements and surface counting

Diethyl (29)

	number	0-3 minutes post injection		17-30 minutes post injection	
		plasma	temple	plasma	temple
normal subjects	11	0.316 ± 0.08	0.188 ± 0.04	0.033 ± 0.009	0.025 ± 0.005
biliary obstruction	5	0.178 ± 0.05	0.040 ± 0.02	0.011 ± 0.004	0.005 ± 0.0001
hepatocellular impairment	23	0.296 ± 0.16	0.187 ± 0.05	0.031 ± 0.01	0.024 ± 0.007

The ratio of the elimination constant from surface counting to the elimination constant from sample measurements, between 17 and 30 minutes, e.g. 0.033 / 0.025, is claimed by the authors to yield an indirect measurement of the fraction removed from blood by the liver (and kidneys?).

6.5. Liver

Weight: MIRD. Phantom 1809 g. Reference man: 1800 g.

Blood content: approximately 15% of liver weight (approximately 250 ml) or

    30% of splanchinc blood volume (294 ml) or

    6% of total blood volume (312 ml)

Tissue composition: parenchymal (polygonal) cells: 65% by number, 90% by weight.

Kupffer's cells	:	35% by number
liver blood flow in		
normal subjects	:	1400 ml (830 - 1890) (30)
cirrhotic patients	:	900 ml (350 - 1520)

Principle behaviour of reagents: A time activity curve obtained from a region of interest situated over liver parenchyma exclusive of larger bile ducts demonstrates a transit type curve with an accumulation segment, a segment of culmination and a segment of reagent elimination.

Parameters evaluated: Visualization of liver by sequential imaging. Hepatic tracer extraction fraction (17). Hepatic uptake rate (17). Time to peak of tracer accumulation in ROI liver. L/H(5)-uptake index: (cpm ROI liver t=5)/ (cpm ROI heart t=5). L/H(10)-uptake index: (cpm ROI liver t=10/(cpm ROI heart t=10) (31,26,32,27). L/H-uptake index, corrected for blood back-ground. Relative tracer concentration (20), counts in ROI liver from an Ida compound at specific point in time devided by counts in ROI liver from Diethylida at same time. Time T max to T max/2. Halftime of tracer washout from liver. 30/ T max-hepatic retention index: (cpm in ROI liver t=30)/(cpm ROI liver at T max). 60/10- Hepatic retention index: (cpm in ROI liver t=60)/(cpm ROI liver at t10). Liver washout index: reciprocal of 60/10 hepatic retention index.

Visualization of liver by sequential imaging: Dimethyl, normal subjects: "within a few minutes following injection". (18). Pyridoxylene glutamate "3-5 minutes post injection" (6).

Hepatic reagent extraction fraction: This parameter is defined as follows: concentration in the femoral artery minus concentration in the hepatic vein divided by the concentration in the femoral artery during constant infusion of

0.3 mg/minute Diethyl-Ida; measured during 3 time intervals: (a) 30-60, (b) 60-90, (c) 90-120 minutes. Results: The arterial concentration increased continuously, the arterio-venous difference remained constant, the extracted fraction therefore decreased (relatively) from 0.56 to 0.42 in one patient, from 0.48 to 0.32 in another patient with steatosis, and in 9 patients with hepatic cirrhosis it ranged between 0.40 and 0.03. Attempts to measure the extraction fraction shortly after the start of the infusion demonstrated widely scattered hepatic extraction efficiencies. The authors attributed this observation to variable rapid mixing. The hepatic uptake rate in µg/minute can be calculated as the arterio-hepaticovenous concentration difference multiplied by the hepatic plasma flow. The hepatic plasma flow was determined from constant infusion of indocyaningreen. The hepatic uptake rate of Diethyl-Ida as a constant infusion of 17 mg/hour remained almost constant between 100-200 µg/minute (except in one patient who revealed an unexplained significant increase (17).

Recorded maximum concentration times post injection from regions of interest over liver not containing major bile ducts:

type of patient	Ida-derivatives used	number	T max minutes	source
normal subjects	Diethyl	17	8.7 ± 1.6	(25)
" "	"	51	6.8 ± 2.7 (3-13 min)	(33)
" "	"	15	7.2 ± 1.9	(34)
			(9 female, 6 male normal subjects)	
" "	"	5	10.5 ± 2.6	(35)
" "	"	20	10.4 ± 3.9	(26)
" "	Trimethyl	5	10.9 ± 2.8	(35)
" "	Diisopropyl	5	13.0	(36)
" "	p-butyl	5	16.2 ± 3.8	(35)
" "	Diisopropyl	20	14.7	(37)
" "	p-isopropyl	20	17.1 ± 4.7	(38)
cirrhosis	Diethyl	15	14.3 ± 5.6	(33)
"	"	8	17.3 ± 2.3	(22)
"	p-isopropyl	8	19.2 ± 2.9	(22)
alcoholic cirrhosis				
no cholestasis		1	10.4	
chronic hepatitis		1	21.2	

alcoholic cirrhosis

cholestasis		1	16.4	
cholangio-carcinoma				
standard procedure				
tube insertion		1	19.2	
obstructive jaundice				
cancer of papilla		1	1.6 (accumulatory failure)	
cholecystectomy	Diethyl	23	12.1 ± 3.7	(34)
cholecystectomy no				
calculi		9	12.5 ± 3.9	(25)
choledocho				
lithiasis	Diethyl	18	7.4 ± 1.7	(34)
without obstruction	Diethyl	10	10.8 ± 2.8	(25)

Liver / Heart uptake index (L/H)

(cpm ROI liver)/(cpm ROI heart)

at t=3 or 5 or 10 minutes post injection

normal patients	Diethyl	20	1.64 ± 0.61(L/H at t=3)	(26)
" "	p-isopropyl	20	1.31 ± 0.41(L/H at t=3)	(26)
cirrhosis	Diethyl	8	1.94 ± 0.39(L/H at t=5)	(37)
"	p-isopropyl	8	1.15 ± 0.33(L/H at t=5)	(37)

Liver/heart (10 minutes) uptake index: (27,39) (see further in text).

Liver/heart (10 minutes) corrected uptake index: Ida counts (ROI liver - HSA counts ROI liver) / (HSA counts ROI liver). This number is an index of net liver uptake corrected for liver blood-pool at 10 minutes, prior to the administration is given to determine the ratio of the liver to heart albumin spaces (S) for later curve correction. Assuming the rate of disappearance of activity from the liver blood-pool is the same as from the heart, the estimated liver blood-pool retention curve was derived by multiplying each point on the heart blood-pool retention curve by the liver/heart albumin space ratio (S) determined with Tc^{99m}-albumin (S/H=LBl).

The estimated liver blood-pool retention curve was then subtracted from the gross liver uptake curve to yield a net liver uptake curve (Grl-LBl=NtL). Cursers in approximately the same location were used in the 1 hour post injection recording to obtain the counts/channel for the liver and heart respectively. To derive the net liver counts/channel/frame at 1 hour, the heart counts/channel were multiplied by the liver/heart albumin space ratio and subtracted from gross liver counts/channel. The difference was then normalized for counting time (27,39). Net cpm ROI liver calculated HSA counts ROI liver. Calculated HSA counts ROI liver = counts ROI heart x S (liver to heart albimun ratio).

Relative tracer concentration: Definition: Counts in ROI liver-parenchyma from an ida-compound at a specific point in time divided by counts in ROI-liver-parenchyma from Diethylida at the same time. The administered doses were checked by comparison with standards (35).

Normal subjects   : N = 5
Trimethyl/diethyl : 0.7
p-butyl-diethyl   : 1,4

Retention index: (cpm ROI liver 30 minutes post injection)/(cpm ROI liver at T max). This number is an index of the fraction retained within liver parenchyma; all authors state that their ROI's do not include bile ducts.

type of subject	Ida-derivatives	number	retention index	source
normal subjects	Diethyl	7	0.60	(31)
" "	"	5	0.60	(35)
" "	Trimethyl	5	0.80	(35)
" "	p-butyl	5	0.90	(35)
" "	Diethyl	20	0.61-0.19	(26)
" "	p-isopropyl	20	0.84-0.12	(26)

Halflive of hepatic reagent elimination: Definition: True halflife estimation from time an activity curve obtained from a ROI liver parenchyma from T max to at least 45 minutes post injection.

	Diethyl-Ida	Diisopropyl-Ida
time to peak	11 minutes	13 minutes

liver wash-out I: 3.6% : 0.55 minutes 7%: 1.42 minutes
             II:96.4% :24.75 minutes 93%:27.72 minutes

L/H (10)- uptake index   (counts ROI liver t = 10)/(counts ROI heart t = 10)

type of subject	number	Ida-derivatives	uncorrected	corrected
normal subjects	20	Diethyl	6.84 – 2.99	7.37 – 3.90
"	20	Diisopropyl	10.27 – 4.37	12.01 – 6.51
"	9	Diisopropyl	12.07 – 2.82	12.80 – 3.12
"	9	p-isobutyl	6.36 – 1.71	6.62 – 3.41
hyperbilirubin-emia 1-5 mg/dl	16	Diethyl	5.14 – 3.73	5.18 – 4.03
"	16	Diisopropyl	7.37 – 3.91	7.66 – 4.20
"	17	Diisopropyl	7.15 – 3.34	6.92 – 3.41
"	17	p-butyl	4.91 – 2.34	4.57 – 2.91
Hyperbilirubin-emia greater than 5 mg/dl	8	Diethyl	0.99 – 0.19	0.29 – 0.11
"	8	Diisopropyl	1.32 – 0.31	0.88 – 0.52
"	7	Diisopropyl	3.19 – 1.63	3.55 – 2.35
"	7	p-butyl	1.65 – 1.05	1.47 – 1.59

T max/2:

Definition: Time interval between the time of maximum count to the time of half the maximum counts in ROI over liver parenchyma; so called T/2 downslope. This is really a linear halftime approximation of hepatic parenchymal tracer elimination corresponding to biliary secretion if biliary obstruction or a storage pattern of bile flow can be ruled out.

type of patient	number	Ida-derivatives	value observed	source
normal subjects	51	Diethyl	15.8 - 6.7 minutes (7-30)	(33)
"	15	"	27.1 - 5.2	(34)
"	17	"	16.4 - 2.0	(25)
"	20	Diisopropyl	22 minutes	(37)
"	10	Diethyl	16 - 20	(24)
"	10	Diethyl, RLL	23.2 - 3.4	(32)
"	10	Diethyl, LLL	22.8 - 5.1	(32)
cirrhosis	8	Diethyl	75.0 - 29.0	(22)
"	8	p-isopropyl	130.0 - 44.0	(22)
"	1	Diethyl	69.7 minutes	(25)
"	30	"	more than 30 minutes	(33)
steatosis	12	"	approximately 50 minutes	(24)
parenchymal liver disease standard procedure chole-cystectomy	42	"	more than 30 minutes 30 =	(32)
cholelithiasis without obstruction	8	"	27.9 - 7.7	(25)
cholelithiasis without obstruction	9	"	26.2 - 4.5	(25)
obstruction	18	"	38.4 - 5.2	(34)

Retention index: The fraction of reagent concentration present at 10 minutes post injection still left in liver at 60 minutes post injection corrected for blood back-ground. Ida counts ROI liver-HSA counts ROI liver at 10 minutes and 60 minutes net cpm = 60/net cpm t = 10. The lower the number the better the compound for the study of hepatobiliary elimination and bile flow.

type of subject	number	Ida-derivatives	retention index
normal subjects	20	Diethyl	0.206
" "	20	Diisopropyl	0.275
" "	7	"	0.283
" "	7	p-butyl	0.806
hyperbilirubinemia			
between 1-5 mg/dl	15	Diethyl	0.507
" "	15	Diisopropyl	0.520
" "	12	"	0.469
" "	12	p-butyl	0.934
hyperbilirubinemia			
greater than 5 mg%	8	Diethyl	1.07
" "	8	Diisopropyl	1.16
" "	7	"	.775
" "	7	p-butyl	1.01
average of all patients	43	Diethyl	.321
" " "	43	Diisopropyl	.396
" " "	26	"	.410
" " "	26	p-butyl	1.01

Liver wash-out index: Definition: The liver wash-out index is obtained by the following relation, which is the reciprocal of the 60/10. Retention index: (cpm in ROI liver at 10 minutes)/(cpm in ROI liver at 60 minutes) from Hernandez and Rosenthall (27,39). This number is an index of biliary secretion; the higher the number the better the compound.

Patients with bilirubin-levels below 1 mg/dl:

number	Ida-derivatives	wash-out index
7	p-butyl	1.24 ± 0.28
7	Diisopropyl	3.53 ± 1.60
20	"	3.63 ± 1.98
20	Diethyl	4.85 ± 4.09

Patients with hyperbilirubinemia of 1 - mg/dl:

12	p-butyl	1.07 ± 0.64
12	Diisopropyl	2.13 ± 1.40
15	"	1.92 ± 1.11
15	Diethyl	1.97 ± 1.56

Patients with hyperbilirubinemia of more than 5 mg/dl:

7	p-butyl	0.50 ± 0.09 values below 1.0 are due
7	Diisopropyl	1.29 ± 0.56 to reference time point of
8	"	0.86 ± 0.28 10 minutes being earlier
8	Diethyl	0.93 ± 0.17 than peak.

Group of all patients listed above:

26	p-butyl	0.99 ± 0.51
26	Diisopropyl	2.44 ± 1.53
43	"	2.52 ± 1.86
43	Diethyl	3.11 ± 3.37

6.6. Gall-bladder, bile ducts

The ICRP-report on reference man states: "The gall-bladder is a sack-like organ which normally stores and concentrates the bile which it receives from the liver by way of the hepatic and cystic ducts".

Dimensions: length: 8 - 12 cm, width 4 - 5 cm

weight: adult male: 10 g, adult female: 8 g

thickness of wall: 1 - 2 mm

shape: conical of pearshaped

volume: 50 - 65 ml (30 - 90 ml at other authors)

Bile flow: gall-bladder bile: 0.13 - 0.2 ml/minute

          liver bile   : 2.6 -15   ml/kg W for 24 hours

          normal range   : 800 - 1000 ml bile per day.

Secretory pressure: 15 - 25 cm H_2O

    Hepatobiliary tracers follow the flow of bile after they have been secreted at the biliary pole of the hepatocytes. In normal subjects two patterns have been observed, a so called excretion pattern and a storage pattern. In the excretion pattern the bile ducts within the liver become scarcely recognizable, tracer passes through the common bile duct into the duodenum before accumulation begins in the gall-bladder. In the storage pattern there is no initial transit of labeled bile into the duodenum, but there is promiment visualization of branching streaks of intrahepatic hyperactivity corresponding to accumulation of tracer in the intrahepatic bile duct. There is also accumulation of tracer in the gall-bladder, if the cystic duct is patent. The excretion pattern is observed about 4 to 5 times more frequently than the storage pattern. Accumulation within the gall-bladder always begins only after an initial lag-time and continues for several hours or until contraction of the gall-bladder is stimulated by cholecystokinin injection or the eating of a test meal.

    <u>Parameters which have been evaluated are:</u>

The time of tracer appearance respectively visualization of gall-bladder.

The frequency of visualization.

An analog recording of accumulation curve.

    <u>Visualization of the gall-bladder:</u> time of reagent appearance.

Normal subjects:

reagent	number	time	sources
Diethylida (fasting	17	7 - 25 minutes	(40)
" (non-fasting)	5	15 - 34 "	(40)
"	51	26.6 ± 24.4 minutes	
		resp. 5 - 120 minutes occasionally	
		later than 110 minutes	(41)
"	15	23.8 ± 5 minutes	(34)
"		10 - 40 minutes	(42)

Cirrhosis:

Diethyl-Ida	15	39.5 ± 32.9 minutes	(41)
"	8	17.0 ± 6.3 "	(22)
p-isopropyl	8	36.0 ±16.5 "	(22)

The frequency of the visualization of the bile ducts:

Normal subjects, Diethyl-Ida:

number 51   left hepatic bile duct visible in 58.8%

            right   "   "   "   "   " 5.8% (41)

The visualization of the common bile duct in:

Normal Subjects:

reagent	number	time	source
Diethyl	51	12 ± 4.5 minutes range 5-25 minutes	(33)
"	15	13.8 ± 12.1 "	(34)
"	17	7.2 ± 2.9 ."	(25)
Dimethyl	12	10 - 20 minutes	(18)
Pyridoxyliden-glutamate		about 10 minutes	(6)
		10 - 15 minutes	(7)

In cholelithiasis without obstruction:

Diethyl	10	8.8 ± 4.8 minutes	(25)

With cholecystectomy, no calculi:

Diethyl	9	9.8 ± 1.9 minutes	(25)

In cirrhosis:

Diethyl	15	18.4 ± 10.4 minutes	(41)

Visualization of the gall-bladder: Pauwels et al (40) never failed to visualize a healthy gall-bladder using Diethyl-Ida in a reliably fasting patient. Two false-positives occured in non-fasting patients using Tc^{99m}-PyG. Matolo et al (43) stressed the importance of a fat free diet to avoid false positive results. The incidence of false-positive results i.e. non-visualization of the gall-bladder in patients with no cholecystitis, appears to be higher with Tc^{99m}-Dihydrothioctic acid (44)

6.7. The intestine

weight:	ICRP:	MIRD PHANTOM
small intestine, wall :	640 g	1044 g
contents :	400 g	
upper large intestine		
wall :	210	209.2
contents :	220	200
lower large intestine		
wall :	160	160.1
contents :	135	136.8

In normal non-fasting patients hepatobiliary reagents appear in the region of the duodenum within 10 - 30 minutes of intravenous injection, usually preceding reagent appearance in the gall-bladder by 10 - 15 minutes. Drainage of reagent containing bile continues for about 1 - 3 hours. Propagation of the reagent along the intestinal tract occurs usually as a bolus. The ascending colon is rarely reached before 4 hours post injection.

The time of appearance in duodenum in normal fasting subjects using Diethyl-Ida has been shown to be variable:

number	time		source
15	16.5 ± 6.5 minutes 5 - 30 minutes ("excretion pattern") observed in 43/51		(41)
51	79.3 ± 49.5 " 25 -150 " ("storage pattern") observed in 8/51		(41)
15	13.8 ± 2.1 "		(34)
18	5 - 37 minutes ("excretion pattern")		(40)
5	ca. 55 minutes ("storage pattern", resp. 10 minutes after gall-bladder stimulation		

In cholelithiasis the values observed with Dietyl-Ida were:

18	14.1 ± 1.8 minutes	(34)

and after cholecystectomy:

number	time	source
23	14.5 + 1.8 minutes	(34)

in cirrhosis, Diethyl-Ida values were:

| 15 | 5 - 55 minutes ("excretion pattern") | |
| | 85 ± 7 minutes ("storage pattern") | (34) |

with Pyridoxylidenglutamate the following values were obtained:

normal subjects	:	20 minutes	(7)
patients (bilirubin 2.8 mg/dl)	: 30 - 180		(45)
patients (bilirubin 11 mg/dl)	: after 24 hours		
patients (bilirubin 12.2 mg/dl)	: no tracer in intestine		

With respect to the residence time in intestinal tract Diethyl administered via a duodenal tube in 7 patients with sequential imaging at 30, 60, 120, 240 and 300 minutes post injection showed that administered activity travelled as a drawn-out bolus through the small bowel between 30 and 240 minutes, was thought to be present in ascending colon by 300 minutes post injection. Clearly identifiable parts of the small bowel could not be distinguished (46)

Activity was observed in the colon in a mixed group of patients: number 10: at 4 hours post injection 2 patients (in the other 8 patients: activity in lower small bowel at 4 hours). With liver transplant patients, number 5: diethyl-ida activity was present in the colon at 24 hours post injection in 3 cases. In the case of Diethyl-Ida in a normal subject colon-activity was seen at 18 hours and in 1 patient with hepatocellular hyperbilirubinemia of 18 mg/dl at 19 hours. The amount of colonic tracer content was distinctly less when evaluated at image interpretation (18)

Intestinal reabsorption: Measurements of Diethyl-Hida concentrations were made in blood and urine together with sequential images of the gall-bladder, up to 5 hours after administering the reagent via an intestinal tube in 7 subjects. No visualization of the gall-bladder was observed and the blood-concentration was 0.004 - 0.69% of the administered dose. The cumulative 4 hours urine excretion was 0.1 - 0.8% of the administered radioactivity (46) Similar measurements in rats gave the same results(42) . Duodeno-gastric reflux was not observed in a group of 51 normal persons (33) but was observed in 10% of a second group of persons (38).

The fraction of the administered dose in bowel using Diethyl-Ida a comparison of the activity in a large anterior region of interest containing bowel was made in 5 patients after oral (via duodenal tube) and intravenous administration. Each patient served as his own standard (fig.2).

Time post injection:	1	2	3	4	5	hours
$\bar{x}$:		11.7	20.4	40.0	59.8	61.6	% administered dose

A fatty meal to stimulate gall-bladder emptying was given after the 3 hours images and frames had been obtained (36)

6.8. Extracellular space

Volume: 20% body weight. Diffusion of Ida-derivatives into and out of extracellular space is expected to take place. The measurement of Diethyl-Ida concentrations in ascitic fluid revealed an increase up to 2 hours post injection and a decrease thereafter which paralleled the decrease in plasma concentration when followed up to 4 hours post injection and confirmed by simultaneous measurement of ^{51}Cr-EDTA in plasma and ascites, which gave identical results.

Surface measurements of activity in the temporal region of the skull: Diethyl monitoring of surface activity measurements of Diethyl-Ida concentrations over the temple have been continously recorded up to 30 minutes post injection. In 11 normal subjects the results obtained were:

between 0- 3 minutes:T/2:3.85 $\pm$ 0.9 minutes k = 0.188 $\pm$ 0.04 / minutes
between 17-30 minutes:T/2:28.1 $\pm$ 6.3 minutes k = 0.025 $\pm$ 0.005/ minutes

In 5 patients with biliary obstruction the values were:

between 0- 3 minutes:T/2:19.7 $\pm$ 7.2 minutes k= 0.040 $\pm$ 0.02   / minutes
between 17-30 minutes:T/2:199 $\pm$ 153 minutes k = 0.005 $\pm$ 0.0001/ minutes

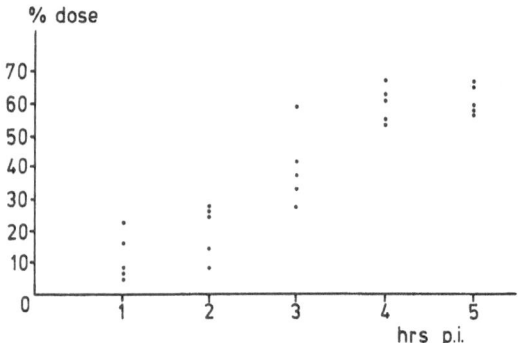

Fig. 2. Hepato biliary Tc^{99m} agents: biodistribution % dose in intestine N-5.

In 23 patients with parenchymal hepatic dysfunction:

between 0- 3 minutes: T/2: 4.04 $\pm$ 1.3 minutes k= 0.187 $\pm$ 0.05 minutes

between 17-30 minutes: T/2: 33.1 $\pm$ 13.3 minutes k= 0.024 $\pm$ 0.007 minutes (29)

Femoral surface activity: In biliary obstruction Diethyl-Ida accumulation curves with a plateau-like culmination at 10 - 30 minutes post injection were observed (29).

6.9. Kidneys and urinary tract.

Weight: In reference man report: 310 g, MIRD phantom: 284.? g. Hepato-biliary reagents visualize the kidneys for a short period of time following intravenous injection. They are excreted in the urine to a variable extent. The degree of urinary excretion appears to depend upon the specific properties of the reagent and the functional status of the liver.

Renal extraction: In six patients, catheters were placed into the femoral artery and the right renal vein. Samples were taken from both. The renal extraction fraction of Tc^{99m} Diethyl-Ida was about 0.07 (range 0.04 - 0.138 which is relatively small. The total renal excretion increases with decreasing hepatic function (17).

Visualization of the kidneys on sequential imaging: In normal subjects with Diethyl-Ida visualisation of the kidneys frequently occured at 5 - 10 minutes post injection disappearing between 20 - 30 minutes (42) Biersack et al (33) observed visualization in normal subjects with Dimethyl-Ida between 5 and 10 minutes post injection but not after 30 minutes and with Diethyl-Ida in 51 patients the kidneys were observed later than 5 minutes in 19.1% of normal subjects, and in no case later than 15 minutes. Pauwels et al (40) also observed no kidney activity after 15 minutes post injection in a series of 22 normal patients. In hepatocellular jaundice (bilirubin 18 mg/dl) with Dimethyl-Ida the renal activity is visible at 1 hour post injection. With hepatocellular jaundice (bilirubin 18 mg/dl), Dimethyl-Ida activity was present within the urinary-bladder 19 hours post injection indicating continuing renal tracer excretion (18).

The cumulative urinary excretion has been measured by a number of investigations at various times post injection:

60 minutes:

normal subjects, Dimethyl-Ida 13.8 ± 2.3% (47)
normal subjects, Diethyl-Ida 10.6 ± 3.0% (47)

90 minutes:

normal subjects: Dimethyl-Ida, number 12: 14.2 ± 1.8 (18)

2 hours:

In patients with cirrhosis, steatosis, Diethyl-Ida, number 6: 5.9%, range:
1.2 - 15 (17).

3 hours:

normal subjects, Diethyl-Ida   number 5: 7.5% (22)
hepatic cirrhosis, Diethyl-Ida   : 8.0 ± 3.5% (22)
hepatic cirrhosis, p-isoprpyl-Ida : 14.9 ± 5.1% (27)

4 hours: (20)

normal subjects, Diethyl-Ida   number 5: 11%
normal subjects, Trimethyl-Ida number 5: 23%
normal subjects, p-butyl-Ida   number 5: 5%

In 4 patients with complete biliary obstruction, Diethyl-Ida excretion was:

(a) 54%, (b) 39%
(c) 52%, (d) 50%

In 1 patient with hepatitis (bilirubin 15 mg/dl), Diethyl-Ida excretion was 74%
and in 5 patients with steatosis (bilirubin 0.3 - 1.4 mg/dl) 9.7%.

24 hours post injection in 6 patients with cirrhosis, steatosis, Diethyl-Ida
excretion was 20%, range 2 - 40% (17)

6.10. Fractions of doses and residence times.

With respect to the percentage accumulated dose in significant-source
regions there is the customary paucity of data in the literature. The results of
measurements of percentage administered dose in blood, urine and intestinal tract
are given in the corresponding sections above.

I have used Tc^{99m} Diethyl-Ida in more than 150 patients. Our routine has
evolved over a period of about 1 year. We believe that very little extra information can be gained after about 4 hours post injection excepting the delayed
images to check for intestinal depots of activity. The following tables

represent an estimation of the time intervals of presence in one of the source regions:

timepoints (hours post injection)	tracer appearance	disappearance
heart	0.01	0.1
liver	0.01	6
duodenum	0.20	1.5
bileducts	0.25	0.5/2
gall-bladder	0.30	stimulated
jejunum	0.5	2
ileum	2	4
upper colon	4	18
lower colon	5	24
kidneys	0.01	0.15
urine-bladder	0.25	24
Times are for Tc^{99m} Diethyl-Ida or Diisopropyl-Ida.		

When the times of throughput were less well known, certain fractions of the administered activity was assumed to decay completely within the following source regions. Since no S-value was available for gall-bladder as a source region the corresponding pancreas value was used as a rough approximation of a "worst case" situation; the assumed fractional dose distribution and the radiation doses from total decay within the source regions are given in the following table:

Fictitious Tc^{99m}-hepatobiliary agent: estimated absorbed radiation doses		
	% dose	rad/mCi
liver	17	0.008
gall-bladder	13.6	0.356
small intestine	13.6	0.097
upper large intestine	13.6	0.199
lower large intestine	27.2	0.464
kidneys	0.5	0.032
urinary-bladder wall	4.5	0.086
ovaries	-	0.075
testes	-	0.008
bone marrow	-	0.030
total body	10.0	0.020

Tc 99m Diethyl-Ida:% dose distribution at 4 hours post injection:

hist. no. of patient	cumulat. urin. excr. (1)	blood-volume (2)	intestin. tract (3)	extracell. space (4)	gall-bladder (liver) (5)
32846	4,5%	2,6%	66,9%	13,2%	12,8%
34998	16,2%	4,0%	54,4%	19,7%	5,7%
35078	13,1%	2,4%	61,5%	11,5%	11,5%
32507	9,5%	3,1%	62,5%	13,4%	11,4%
35760	10,1%	2,7%	53,6%	10,4%	23,2%
$\bar{x}$	10,7%	3,0%	59,8%	13,6%	12,9%

(1): (concentration in urine x volume voided up to 4 hours post injection) / injected activity

(2): (concentration in whole blood at 4 hours x 7% w) / injected activity

(3): external abdominal counts at 4 hours post injection, dose x 100/external abdominal counts after oral dose

(4): (concentration is plasma at 4 hours x 20% w) / injected activity

(5): 100% - (sum of % dose in urine, blood, intestine and extracellular space)

Based on my own % dose measurements in 5 patients (see text) I have attempted to balance the fractional activity distribution at 4 hours post injection. The results are given in the above table.

The estimated absorbed radiation doses to various tissues of an average adult patient from intravenous injections of either 5 or 15 mCi Tc^{99m}-ida injection as estimated by a manufacturer for patients with normal liver function and for those with obstructive jaundice are given below:

Tc^{99m}-Dimethyl-Ida: estimated absorbed radiation doses

| | rads / 5 mCi | | rads / 15 mCi | |
| | normal | obstructive | normal | obstructive |
tissue	liver	jaundice	liver	jaundice
liver	0.20	0.23	0.59	0.68
small intestine	1.62	0.11	4.86	0.32
upper large				
intestine wall	4.14	0.17	12.41	0.51
lower large				
intestine wall	4.58	0.22	13.73	0.65
kidneys	0.17	0.14	0.51	0.41
bladder-wall				
4-8 hours void	0.62	1.53	1.86	4.59
ovaries	0.91	0.12	2.73	0.36
testes	0.07	0.07	0.20	0.20
whole body	0.16	0.06	0.47	0.17

The methodology of absorbed dose determination for Tc^{99m}-Dihydrothiotic acid was discussed by Vanek and Brookeman (49) and the kinetics and dosimetry in general of radiopharmaceuticals utilized in evaluating liver, gall-bladder and spleen by Spencer et al (50)

6.11. Discussion

Biliary elimination is an important excretory pathway for both endogenous lipophylic substances, such as bilirubin, hormones, and a great many drugs, chemicals and their metabolites. Hepatocytes excrete 4 groups of substances: the bile acids (responsible for the bile acids dependent bile flow), organic anions (including conjugated bilirubin and dyes such as BSP, indocyanine green etc), organic cations and neutral substances, e.g. cardiac glyosides, all depending upon the bile acid independent bile flow. These 4 groups are probably excreted by different pathways since no competition for biliary excretion has been described among them, although this has been observed within each group.

The data compiled from the literature and listed above reveal subtle, albeit distinct differences of degree in the principle pattern of biological distribution of hepatobiliary Tc^{99m}-Ida-derivatives. The differences are found in the degree of hepatic uptake, in the speed of secretion into bile, in blood clearance and urinary elimination. They are due to specific properties of the compounds on one hand and due to impairment of hepatocyte function in various disease states on the other.

These differences can better be appreciated in an analog way than by tedious scrutiny of the above numbers. The visual evanuation of follow-up studies can show the gradual restitution of hepatocytic dysfunction.

The intriguing question which follows is: How would a depression of hepato-biliary function affect the behaviour and relative differences of the other tracer as Trimethyl-Ida, Diisopropyl-Ida, p-isopropyl-Ida. The Diethyl-Ida studies reveal delayed hepatobiliary transfer, but adequate visualization of the bile-ducts demonstrating open pathways. The p-butyl-Ida studies show better hepatic uptake but do not visualize the bile ducts. This again illustrates the results of the indices. P-Butyl-Ida reaches its maximum concentration in the liver distinctly later and leaves the liver more slowly than Diethyl-Ida and this the more so in cirrhosis, toxic hepatopathy or hepatocytic impairment secondary to partial or total obstruction.

There is an interrelationship between hepatic uptake and concentration in bile. It is trivial to point out that bile cannot contain more reagent than was present in the liver, before secretion began, but bile can contain very much less reagent (radioactivity/ml) dependent upon the speed at which it leaves the hepatocytes, i.e. biliary secretion. The downslope of hepatic paren-chymal reagent content is due to and represents biliary secretion. Given the same amount of various reagents within the liver the downslopes of their elimination from liver into non-obstructed bile ducts are proportional to their concentrations in bile (making the reasonable assumption that the rate of bile production is fairly constant). Given the same reagent in a patient at different points in time during the course of some hepatobiliary disorder the downslope will again represent biliary secretion, whereas uptake is the result of liver blood flow and extraction efficiency.

The following generalizations can be made (from the compiled numbers and sequential imaging):

a) The biological distribution of a Tc^{99m} labeled Ida-derivative depends strongly upon the functional state of the hepatocyte.

b) The same kind and degree of impairment of the hepatocytes will affect differently the hepatic uptake of a Ida-derivative, i.e. the fraction of administered radioactivity entering hepatic parenchyma per unit time, e.g. the uptake of Diethyl-Ida may be depressed distinctly more than that of Parabutyl-Ida ·in hepatocyte impairment.

c) The same kind and degree of impairment e.g. cholangitis, hepatopathy will affect differently the biliary secretion of an Ida-derivative, i.e. the rate at which this compound leaves the hepatocytes; the rate of secretion may became so low that the resultant radioactivity in bile will be insufficient for imaging.

d) Hepatocyte impairment either prolongs the intrahepatic time course thus lowering biliary secretion or diminishes biliary secretion thus prolonging the intrahepatic residence time. This occurs to a lesser degree with Diethyl-Ida of Diisopropyl-Ida than with Parabutyl-Ida.

e) Given the same downslope the higher the hepatic parenchymal uptake the better, since more radioactivity is likely to reach the bile ducts or the intestinal tract.

f) The selection of parameters requires clarification of the aim of comparative evaluation of hepatobiliary reagents. To what end, for what purposes, should the agent under consideration be evaluated. The following applications of hepatobiliary tracers can be envisioned. The parameters studied should be unified, so that comparison of published data will become possible. Diethyl-Ida appears to be known best and is used as the yardstick which the others are evaluated. (fig.1).

(1) = measurement of effective hepatic plasma flow

(2) = measurement of global liverfunction (and its follow up during the course of a therapeutic regime)

(3) = estimation of the relative contributions to liver blood flow from the hepatic artery and portal vein

(4) = assessment of differences in regional liver function

(5) = static imaging of liver parenchyma

(6) = imaging (and, if possible quantification) of biliary secretion, bile flow, biliary stasis, intrahepatic cholestasis

(7) = imaging of biliary motility and dyskinesia

(8) = measurement of urinary excretion as a measurement of impairment of hepatic uptake

(9) = imaging (and possibly quantification) of duodeno-gastric or jejuno-gastric reflux, of biliodigestive or intestinal tracer propagation.

The parameters of interest in characterizing quantitatively the principle pattern of biological distribution of hepatobiliary tracers are:

The degree of hepatic uptake i.e. the fraction of administered activity time.

The extent of biliary secretion.

The speed of hepatic throughput.

The cumulative intestinal elimination.

The cumulative urinary excretion.

The retention in blood and total body.

Unfortunately these parameters are very difficult or even impossible to measure. Therefore most authors use either indices or some other equivalent of the measurement. Significant source regions to be considered in the dosimetry of Tc^{99m} labeled hepatobiliary reagents in humans are the gall-bladder, the various parts of the intestinal tract, the urinary bladder, the liver, the kidneys and the blood with the rest of the body. The fractional distribution and the residence times in the source regions of each of these reagents are not known with a sufficient degree of certainty. Reliable dosimetry does not seem possible as yet, excepting estimations using reasonable assumptions. The radiation dose from a Tc^{99m}-Ida-derivative to a patient with hepatobiliary impairment will be the lower the more readily the kidneys compensate for the diminished hepatobiliary elimination.

REFERENCES

1. Burns D, Marzilli L, Sowa D, Bauem D, Wagner Jr H, Relationship between molecular structure and biliary excretion of Technetium-99m Hida and Hida analogs (abstract) J. nucl. Med. 18:624, 1977.

2. Wistow BW, Subramanian G, Van Heertum RL, Henderson RW, Gagne GM, Hall RC, McAfee JG, An evaluation of 99mTc-labeled hepatobiliary agents. J. nucl. Med. 18:455, 1977.

3. Tonkin AK, DeLand FH, Dihydrothioctic acid: a new polygonal cell imaging agent (abstract) J. nucl. Med. 15:539, 1974.

4. Lin TH, Kentigan A, Winchell HS, A ^{99m}Tc-labeled replacement for ^{131}I-Rose Bengal in liver and biliary tract studies. J. nucl. Med. 15:613, 1974.

5. Baker RJ, Bellen JC, Ronai PM, 99mTc-pyridoxylideneglutamate: a new rapid cholescintigraphic agent. J. nucl. Med. 15:476, 1974.

6. Baker RJ, Bellen JC, Ronai PM, Technetium pyridoxilideneglutamate: a new hepatobiliary radiopharmaceutical. I. Experimental aspects. J. nucl. Med. 16:720, 1975.

7. Ronai PM, Baker RJ, Bellen JC, Technetium 99m pyridoxylidene glutamate, a new hepatobiliary radiopharmaceutical. II. Clinical aspects. J. nucl. Med. 16:728, 1975.

8. Poulose KP, Eckelman WC, Reba RC, Evaluation of 99mTc-pyridoxylideneglutamate for the differential diagnosis of jaundice. Clin. Nucl. Med. 1:70, 1976.

9. Fotopoulos A, Evaluation of 99mTc-pyridoxalphenylalanine as a hepatobiliary imaging agent. Part. F. Experimental studies. J. nucl. Med. 18:1189, 1977.

10. Papadimitriou A, Fotopoulos C, Koutoulidis C, Chiotelis E, Tountas C, Evaluation of Tc99m pyridoxal phenyldanine as a hepatobiliary agent. Port 2. Clinical tests. J. nucl. Med. 18:1194, 1977.

11. Fritzberg AR, Lyster DM, Dolphin DH, 99mTc-Bioquin-7 CA, a potential new hepatobiliary scanning agent. J. nucl. Med. 17:907, 1976.

12. Krishnamurthy GT, Tubis M, Endow JS, Blahol WS, Tc-pencillamine, a new radio-pharmaceutical for cholescintigraphy (abstract) J. nucl. Med. 13:447, 1972.

13. Fliegel G, Pewanjee MK, Holman BL, Davis MA, Treves S, ^{99m}Tc tetracycline as a kidney and gall-bladder imaging agent. Radiology 110:407, 1974.

14. Yeh SH, Delahay JE, Kriss JP, Tc 99m labelled toluidine blue O for liver scintillography. Int. J. Appl. Radiat. 19:885, 1968.

15. Loberg MD, Fields AI, Chemical Structure of Technetium-99m-labeled N-(e, 6-dimethylphenylcarbamoylmethyliminodiacetic acid (Tc-HIDA). J. of Appl. Rad. Isot. 29:167, 1978.

16. ICRP,23, Report of the task group on reference man. Oxford, Pergamon press 1974.

17. Hendriksen HJ, Winkler K, Hepatobiliäre Funktionsszintigraphie mit IDA-derivaten. In: Proceedings of the symposium of North-Rhine Westphalian Society of Nuclear Medicine, April 1978, Bonn. Biersack HJ, Mahlstedt J (eds), Darmstadt, G-I-T/E Giebler, 1978.

18. Ryan J, Cooper M, Loberg M, Harvey E, Sikorski S, Technetium-99m-labeled N-(2,6 dimethylpheylcarbamoylmethyl) iminodiacetic acid (Tc-99m HIDA: a new radiopharmaceutical for hepatobiliary imaging studies. J. nucl. Med. 18:995, 1977.

88

19. Passath A, Leb G, Ergebnisse der Leberszintigraphie mit einer neuen Kolloid-substanz (99mTc-Sn-Antipyrin ^{R}D 77 1268) im Vergleich mit 99mTc-Sn-Phytat, 18, 79. Nukl. Med. 18:79, 1979.

20. Fueger GF, Unpublished data, 1977.

21. Fueger GF, Unpublished data, 1978.

22. Dudzak R, Kletter K, Angelberger P, Frischauf H, Comparison of two different biliary agents in healthy subjects and in patients with liver diseases. Eur. J. Nucl. Med. 4:365, 1979.

23. Dudzak R, Angelberger P, Kletter K, Wagner-Löffler M, Ferencsi P, Frischauf H, Comparison of 99mTc-Diethylida with 99mTc-Parabutylida in jaundiced patients. In:IAEA, SM 247 - 153, Proceedings of the IAEA symposium on medical radionuclide imaging, Heidelberg, September 1980.

24. Bengoa J, Ritschard J, Donath A, Szintigraphie hepatobiliäre: rest fonction-nel. Schweiz. med. Wschr. 108:1896, 1978.

25. Joseph K, Mahlstedt J, Welcke U, Pries HH, Hepatobiliäre Funktionsszinti-graphie (HBFS) mit Hepatobida. NucComp. 1:20, 1977.

26. Reichelt HG, Nuklearmedizinische Leber- und Gallenwegsdiagnostik mit dem hepatotropen, cholophilen Radiopharmakon 99mTc-Diäthyl-IDA (EHIDA). NucComp. 9:18, 1978.

27. Hernandez M, Rosenthall L, A cross-over study of the kinetics of 99mTc-labeled Diethyl- and Diisopropyl-IDA. Clin. Nucl. Med. 5:352, 1980.

28. Tongendorff J, Raithel E, Büll U, Grunst J, Trumm F, Scherer R, Die Wertig-keit der hepatobiliären Funktionsszintigraphie mit 99mTc-Diäthyl-IDA. Nucl. Med. 17:30, 1978.

29. Passath A, Leb G, Möglichkeiten in der Differentialdiagnose zwischen Paren-chym- und Verschlussikterus mit 99mTc-Hida durch Auswertung von Funtions-parametern. Nukl. Med. 19:127, 1980.

30. Vetter H, Studies of hepatic circulation, function and morphology. In: Radioisotopes in medical diagnosis, Belcher EH, Vetter H (eds), London, Butterworth, 1971.

31. Pors Nielsen S, Trap-Jensen J, Lindenberg J, Lykkegard Nielsen M, Hepato-biliary scintigraphy and hepatography with Tc-99m diethyl-acetanilido-imino-diacetate in obstructive jaundice. J. nucl. Med. 19:452, 1978.

32. Cox PH, Tjen HSLM, Van der Pompe WB, The clinical value of 99mTc-labelled Diethyl-acetanilido-imino-diacetate complex for dynamic studies of hepato-biliary function. NucComp. 9:67, 1978.

33. Biersack JJ, Breuel HP, Thelen M, Winkler C, Beurteilungskriterien der hepatobiliären Funktionsszintigraphie mit 99m-Tc-markiertem Diäthyl-IDA. Fortschr. Röntgenstr. 130:689, 1979.

34. Kroiss A, Peschl L, Kogelbauer G, Stellamor K, Neumayr A, Hepatobiliäre Diagnostik mit 99mTc-hepatobida. Leber, Magen, Darm 9:107, 1979.

35. Fueger GF, Dittrich G, Diethyl, Trimethyl and p-butyl-derivatives of 99m-Tc hepato-imino-diacetic acid in 5 volonteers and 5 patients with hepato-biliary disease. In: Progress in Radiopharmacology, Vol. I. Cox PH (ed), Amsterdam, Elsevier/North-Holland Biomedical Press, 1979.

36. Fueger GF, Unpublished data, 1980.

37. Cox PH, Unpublished data, personal communication, 1980.

38. Reichelt HG, Langenberg G, Löhlein D, Hepato-biliäre Sequenzszintigraphie in prä- und postoperativer Oberbauchdiagnostik. Chirurg 48:583, 1977.

39. Hernandez M, Rosenthall L, A cross-over study comparing the kinetics of 99m-Tc-labeled Diisopropyl and P-Butyl IDA analogs in patients. Clin. Nucl. Med. 5:159, 1980.

40. Pauwels S, Steels M, Piret L, Beckers C, Clinical evaluation of Tc-99m-Diethyl-IDA in hepatobiliary disorders. Nucl. Med. 19:783, 1978.

41. Biersack JJ, Breuel HP, Thelen M, Winkler C, Beurteilungskriterien der hepatobiliären Funktionsszintigraphie mit 99mTc-markiertem Diäthyl-IDA. Fortschr. Röntgenstr. 130:689, 1979.

42. Tjen HSLM, Cholescintigraphy Ph.D. Thesis, University of Utrecht, The Netherlands (in English), 1979.

43. Matolo NM, Stadalnik RC, Wolfman EF, Hepatobiliary scanning using 99mTc-Pyridoxylidenglutamate. Amer. J. Surg. 133:116, 1977.

44. Eikman EA, Cameron JL, Colman M, Radioactive tracer techniques in the diagnosis of acute cholestitis. J. nucl. Med. 14:393, 1973.

45. Lubin E, Rachima M, Oren V, Weininger J, Trumper J, Korenitzky I, Rechnic Y, Tc99m Pyridoxylidene Glutamate in jaundiced patients. J. nucl. Med. 19:24, 1978.

46. Stöffler G, Holzer H, Chahbazi H, Fueger GF. In: Hepatobiliäre Funktionsszintigraphie mit IDA-Derivaten. Proceedings of the symposium of North-Rhine Westphalian Society of Nuclear Medicine, April 1978, Bonn. Biersack HJ, Mahlstedt J (eds), Darmstadt, G-I-T/E Giebler, 1978.

47. Welcke U, Hepatobiliäre Funktionsszintigraphie mit IDA-Derivaten. Proceedings of the symposium of North-Rhine Westphalian Society of Nuclear Medicine, April 1978, Bonn, Biersack HJ, Mahlstedt J (eds), Darmstadt, G-I-T/E Giebler, 1978.

48. Klingensmith WC, Fritzberg AR, Koep LJ, Comparison of Tc-99m Diethyl-imino-diacetic acid and 1-131 Rose Bengal for Hepatobiliary Studies in Liver-transplant patients: concise communication. J. nucl. Med. 20:314, 1979.

49. Vanek KN, Brookeman VA, Methodology of absorbed dose determinations for a new hepatobiliary imaging agent (99mTc-DHTA). In: Radiopharmaceutical dosimetry symposium, Cloutier RJ, Coffey JL, Snyder WS, Watson EE (eds), Publication (FDA) Washington, 1976.

50. Spencer RP, Hosian F, Spitznagle LA, Kinetics and dosimetry of radiopharmaceuticals utilized in evaluating liver, gall-bladder and spleen. In: Radiopharmaceutical dosimetry symposium, Cloutier RJ, Coffey WS, Snyder WS, Watson EE (eds), Publication (FDA) Washington, 1976.

7. FUNCTIONAL LIVER DISEASE

P.H. COX, H.S.L.M. TJEN

7.1. INTRODUCTION

The use of Technetium-ida derivatives for the clinical diagnosis of liver disease and Diethyl-ida in particular has been reported in some 150 publications since 1977. Much of this information has been reviewed in bookform (1,2, 3,4) and it is not our intention to inventarize this further in the clinical section of this work. In this and succeeding chapters the clinical use of Diethyl-ida will be illustrated on the basis of the authors individual experience. Functional liver disease may manifest itself as single and multiple foci or uniformly disseminated throughout the liver. The use of Diethyl-ida cholescintigraphy coupled with time activity curves and functional images to differentiate these conditions will be discussed in this chapter. Functional imaging as such is discussed in chapter 12.

7.2. Cholescintigraphy in non-obstructive disease

In this series patients with hyper bilirubinaemia were investigated; bile-duct obstruction could not be demonstrated by clinical investigations.
38 patients with jaundice due to parenchymal disease were studied. In 28 patients the diagnosis was confirmed by transcutaneous liver biopsy; in all other patients the diagnosis was confirmed by laparoscopy, operation or post mortem investigation. The classification of these patients is shown in table 1. In the serial scintigrams of 27 patients cholescintigraphy showed a normal intestinal excretion. In the other 11 patients there was delayed excretion. All but two patients with delayed intestinal excretion showed bilirubin values between 217 and 365 μmol/l. Two patients with delayed intestinal excretion had relative low bilirubin values, respectively 32 and 86 μmol/l. Both were shown to suffer from a serious alcoholic hepatitis; in these patients the colloid liver scintigram also showed poor accumulation of colloid in the liver and enhanced accumulation in the RES of spleen and bone marrow.

Table 1. Classification of patients with jaundice due to parenchymal
disease

no. patients	diagnosis
11	acute viral hepatitis
8	drug induced hepatitis
6	alcoholic hepatitis
5	aspecific, reactive hepatitis
3	chronic persistent hepatitis
3	chronic active hepatitis
2	cirrhosis

Table 2 shows the biochemical parameters for each group of patients as
related to the excretion pattern on the serial scintigram. In some patients
the cholescintigraphic investigation was not performed in an early stage of
the illness, because these patients were admitted at a later stage. Time activity curves and functional images for the right and left liver lobes of the
patients investigated are shown in table 3 and compared with total bilirubin
values and intestinal excretion patterns on the serial scintigrams. In 9
patients no time activity curves and functional images could be obtained,
during the 45 minutes in which the investigation was performed only blood-
pool activity was observed. In all these patients intestinal activity was
visible 24 hours after administration of the reagent.

The average maximum uptake time was 13.6 minutes for the right liver lobe
and 15.6 minutes for the left liver lobe. 8 patients showed abnormal upslope
images in spite of normal time activity curves for the related liver lobes
(no. 4,5,13,16,24,30,31,32). In 8 patients there was a slight delay in the
maximum uptake time, for the left and/or the right liver lobe (no. 3,14,15,28,
29,32,36,37); however the upslope image was described as normal.

In 7 patients the time activity curves show a normal excretion for both
liver lobes. In 2 patients there was a normal excretion time for 1 lobe (no.34,
37). Abnormal downslope images were found in spite of normal curves in 8
patients (no. 2,5,7,17,24,26,29,35).

All remaining pathological excretion curves showed delayed patterns:
continuously ascending curves or curves that reach a plateau were not seen.
In addition to biochemical blood analyses in these patients 82 other investigations, encompassing 9 different diagnostic procedures, were performed to

	total bilirubin μmol/l	direct bilirubin μmol/l	alkaline phosphatase mU/ml	S.G.O.T. mU/ml	S.G.P.T. mU/ml	intestinal excretion
acute viral hepatitis	259	165	262	2100	2170	D
	28	-	56	27	96	N
	154	86	157	360	1040	N
	77	48	119	76	124	N
	32	10	181	60	310	N
	217	119	369	1250	1802	D
	50	21	115	62	325	N
	359	232	260	600	756	D
	214	146	238	720	1230	D
	74	42	185	37	170	N
	140	65	169	149	142	N
drug induced hepatitis	36	13	94	93	228	N
	222	110	185	215	330	D
	117	59	178	650	1380	N
	139	67	147	138	148	N
	34	20	787	43	63	N
	26	11	317	203	430	N
	260	168	242	690	1140	D
	365	304	220	628	630	D
alcoholic hepatitis	18	5	76	21	13	N
	103	21	82	24	17	N
	86	52	147	155	83	D
	30	12	121	30	14	N
	32	20	228	112	17	D
	93	40	125	74	20	N
aspecific hepatitis	42	16	263	31	60	N
	66	27	294	13	16	N
	24	5	164	42	122	N
	18	8	134	83	130	N
	167	77	466	129	536	N
chronic persistent hepatitis	78	-	78	650	518	N
	55	16	222	158	207	N
	69	28	600	54	215	N
chronic active hepatitis	264	128	302	1020	900	D
	108	32	86	276	207	N
	21	4	116	146	35	N
cirrhosis	19	2	65	34	28	N
	289	126	195	239	100	D

Table 2. Biochemical parameters of 38 jaundiced patients with various paren-chymal liver disease in comparison to intestinal excretion of Diethyl-ida.
N= normal. D= delayed.

93

	patients no.	total bilirubin µmol/l	intestinal excretion	T-max right	T-max left	T-$\frac{1}{2}$ right	T-$\frac{1}{2}$ left	Upslope right	Upslope left	Downslope right	Downslope left
	1.	259	D	BPA		BPA		BPA		BPA	
	2.	28	N	12	13	23	27	N	N	A	A
acute	3.	154	N	15	25	L	L	N	A	A	A
viral	4.	77	N	12	12	L	L	A	N	A	A
	5.	32	N	10	11	26	22	N	A	A	A
hepatitis	6.	217	D	BPA		BPA		BPA		BPA	
	7.	50	N	8	12	20	18	N	N	N	A
	8.	359	D	BPA		BPA		BPA		BPA	
	9.	214	D	BPA		BPA		BPA		BPA	
	10.	74	N	13	14	L	L	N	N	A	A
	11.	140	N	17	19	L	L	A	A	A	A
	12.	36	N	12	9	9	25	N	N	N	A
drug	13.	222	D	9	15	L	L	A	A	A	A
induced	14.	117	N	15	21	L	L	N	N	N	A
	15.	139	N	14	14	L	L	N	N	A	A
hepatitis	16.	34	N	14	16	L	L	A	A	A	A
	17.	26	N	7	12	30	31	N	N	A	A
	18.	260	D	BPA		BPA		BPA		BPA	
	19.	365	D	BPA		BPA		BPA		BPA	
	20.	18	N	12	9	L	L	N	N	A	N
alcoholic	21.	103	N	25	25	L	L	A	A	A	A
hepatitis	22.	96	D	BPA		BPA		A	A	A	A
	23.	30	N	12	14	L	L	N	N	A	A
	24.	32	D	14	17	21	27	A	A	A	A
	25.	93	N	10	9	L	L	A	A	A	A
	26.	42	N	10	14	30	25	N	N	A	A
aspecific	27.	66	N	14	19	L	L	A	A	A	A
hepatitis	28.	24	N	20	21	L	L	N	N	A	A
	29.	19	N	25	12	30	29	N	N	A	A
	30.	167	N	12	15	L	L	A	A	A	A
chronic	31.	78	N	18	11	L	L	A	A	A	A
persistent	32.	55	N	15	11	L	L	N	A	A	A
hepatitis	33.	69	N	11	14	30	27	N	N	A	A
chronic	34.	264	D	BPA		BPA		BPA		BPA	
active	35.	109	N	15	19	L	27	A	A	A	A
hepatitis	36.	21	N	20	26	L	L	N	N	A	A
cirrhosis	37.	19	N	11	19	29	L	N	N	N	A
	38.	289	D	BPA		BPA		BPA		BPA	

Table 3. Computer data of 38 jaundiced patients with parenchymal liver disease in comparison to total bilirubin values and intestinal excretion in serial scintigrams.
N= normal. D= delayed. L= lengthened. BPA= blood-pool activity. A= abnormal.
Right= right liver lobe. Left= left liver lobe. T max and T$\frac{1}{2}$ are in minutes.

establish whether jaundice was caused by obstruction or parenchymal disease
(see table 4).

Table 4. Investigations in 38 patients with jaundice due to parenchymal
disease: frequency of visualization of liver and biliary tract

diagnostic investigation	no. patients	visualization of liver and biliary tract	
		success	failure
abdominal plain film	15	-	-
oral cholecystography	8	3	5
intravenous cholangio-graphy	11	10	1
percutaneous transhepatic cholangiography	1	0	1
endoscopic cholangio-graphy	1	1	
colloid liver scinti-graphy	13	13	0
ultra sound study	5	5	-
laparoscopy	1	1	-
transcutaneous liver biopsy	28	28	-

In 2 patients abdominal plain film showed concrements in the right upper
abdomen. In the other patients no abnormalities were found. In patients where
oral cholecystography failed, bilirubin values varied from 18 - 108
IVC failed in a patient with a bilirubin value of 108   In 1 patient
intravenous cholangiography could not be performed because of allergy to the
contrast agent. Percutaneous transhepatic cholangiography failed because no
bile-ducts could be visualized.

The contribution which most investigations make to the diagnosis of
jaundice caused by parenchymal disease is that they help to exclude obstruction.
In 10 patients oral cholecystography and intravenous cholangiography showed no
abnormality. In 3 patients there was clearly excretion of the contrast material
by the kidneys when intravenous cholangiography was performed: no obstruction
in the common bile-duct could be demonstrated so that under these conditions
the diagnosis of parenchymal disease was suspected. In 4 patients colloid liver

scintigraphy showed uptake of the radiopharmaceutical by the RES of bone marrow and spleen and in 3 patients a scintigram with a mottled aspect was obtained. Both patterns were suspect for parenchymal disease of the liver. Table 5 shows the findings of the various investigations together with the frequency of correct diagnosis of parenchymal disease.

Table 5. Investigation in 38 jaundiced patients; frequency of findings and frequency of agreement in diagnosis

diagnostic investigation	no. patients	normal	obstruction	parenchymal disease	correct diagnosis
oral cholecysto-graphy	9	3			-
intravenous cholangio-graphy	11	7		3	3
percutaneous trans-hepatic cholangio-graphy	1			1	1
endoscopic cholangio-graphy	1	1			-
colloid liver scinti-graphy	13	6		7	7
ultrasound study	5	3	2		-
laparoscopy	1	1			-
transcutaneous liver biopsy	28		1		27
cholescintigraphy	38	0	0	38	38

Ultra sound investigation demonstrated dilated bile-ducts in 2 patients (table 3 no. 18 and 34) but liver biopsy could not confirm these findings. Percutaneous transhepatic cholangiography did not visualize bile-ducts. This may be due to non-dilated bile-ducts. The final diagnosis in this patient was drug induced hepatitis (table 3 no. 19). In 1 patient liver biopsy showed patterns which were suspect for extrahepatic obstruction (table 3 no.27). However this could not be confirmed by laparoscopy or endoscopic colangiography.

Laparotomy was performed in 2 patients with suspicion of bile-duct obstruction. No obstruction could be demonstrated but during operation parenchymal involvement was confirmed. In both patients cholescintigraphic patterns were suspect for parenchymal disease.

7.3. Discussion

The results of the study revealed the following patterns of cholescintigraphy in patients with jaundice due to parenchymal liver disease.

Serial scintigraphy:

- intestinal excretion of the radiopharmaceutical was observed in all patients
  suffering from parenchymal liver disease
- normal intestinal excretion was observed in 71% of the patients studied
- delayed intestinal excretion was observed in 29%

Patients with a normal intestinal excretion showed a slight persistence of
blood-pool activity in 33% of the total. Intrahepatic bile-ducts were visible
in 63% of this group of patients. Patients with a delayed intestinal excretion
showed a relatively good liver visualization with persistence of a slight blood-
pool activity in 18% and a poor liver visualization with persistence of high
blood-pool activity was observed in 82%.

No additional information could be obtained with the computer in 24% of
the patients studied. Time activity curves obtained from the 2 patients with a
delayed intestinal excretion and persistence of slight blood-pool activity
showed:

- marginally normal T max for both liver lobes
- normal $T\frac{1}{2}$ for both liver lobes in one of the patients studied
- lengthened $T\frac{1}{2}$ for both liver lobes in one of the patients studied

Functional images generated in patients with delayed intestinal excretion
show that in all cases there was a disturbed uptake and excretion phase for both
liver lobes. Time activity curves obtained from patients with a normal intestinal excretion of the radiopharmaceutical showed:

- normal T max for both liver lobes in 44% of the patients studied
- delayed T max for both liver lobes in 30%
- delayed T max for only the right lobe in 22%
- delayed T max for only the left liver lobe in 4%
- normal $T\frac{1}{2}$ for both liver lobes in 31% of the patients studied
- lengthened $T\frac{1}{2}$ for both liver lobes in 63%
- lengthened $T\frac{1}{2}$ for only the left liver lobe in 3%
- lengthened $T\frac{1}{2}$ for only the right liver lobe in 3%

Functional images generated in all the patients studied with normal intestinal excretion, revealed the following patterns:

- disturbed uptake and excretion phase for both liver lobes was observed in 30%
- disturbed uptake phase for one of the lobes and disturbed excretion phase for

both liver lobes was observed in 15%

- normal uptake phase for both liver lobes and disturbed excretion phase for
  both liver lobes was observed in 37%
- disturbed excretion phase for only the left liver lobe was observed in 18%

In 26% of the patients studied a normal intestinal excretion with normal patterns on the time activity curves were observed. All these patients showed abnormal functional images. In 28% of the patients with normal or delayed intestinal excretion there were normal functional images in spite of abnormal patterns in the corresponding time activity curve.

Parenchymal disturbance could be suspected on the serial scintigram if there was a delayed intestinal excretion of the radiopharmaceutical with poor liver visualization and persistent high blood-pool activity. In this series of patients studied intrahepatic cholestasis as the causative agent for the jaundice could be diagnosed on the serial scintigram only in 24%. A slight persistent blood-pool activity in patients with normal intestinal excretion and in patients with delayed intestinal excretion was also indicative of parenchymal disease, although these patterns can also appear in patients with obstructive disease. Computer data in all patients with parenchymal disease of the liver and jaundice showed normal or abnormal patterns of time activity curves but all had normal functional images.

Parenchymal disease could be concluded in this group from the computer data when the typical patterns of time activity curves of obstructed patients were absent, when both time activity curves and functional images were disturbed and especially in patients with normal time activity curves and disturbed functional images. When serial scintigram patterns and computer data were combined the success rate in diagnosing intrahepatic cholestasis as the cause for jaundice was 100%. In comparison the success rate in diagnosing parenchymal disease was for intravenous cholangiography 27%, for liverscintigraphy 54% and for liver biopsy 96%. Ultrasound could not diagnose parenchymal disease in the patients studied.

7.4. Case histories

Les us now consider some individual case histories to illustrate this group of patients.

Case no. 1

A 86-year old female was admitted because of biochemical liver function disturbances and a tumour in the abdomen.

Laboratory findings:	total bilirubin 19 umol/l, direct reacting bili-rubin 2 μmol/l, alkaline phosphatase 65 mU/ml, SGOT 34 mU/ml, SGPT 28 mU/ml.
Colloid liverscintigraphy:	normal findings
Cholescintigraphy serial scintigraphy (fig. 1-23):	good visualization of the liver, no persistent blood-pool activity, normal bile-ducts and gall-bladder visibility. There was also a normal intestinal excretion of the radiopharmaceutical.
Time activity curves: (fig. 1-24)	normal uptake and excretion patterns for the right lobe and a delayed uptake and excretion for the left liver lobe
Functional images: (fig. 1-25)	normal uptake and excretion phase for the right liver lobe and a disturbed uptake and excretion phase for the left liver lobe.
Conclusion:	no bile-duct obstruction, disturbance of liver parenchyma from the left liver lobe
Liver biopsy:	during operation from both right and left liver lobes, showed no abnormality in the right lobe and cirrhosis in the left lobe.

Case no. 2

A 20-year old male was admitted with a suspicion of acute viral hepatitis.

Laboratory findings:	total bilirubin 32 μmol/l, direct reacting bili-rubin 10 μmol/l, alkaline phosphatase 181 mU/ml, SGOT 60 mU/ml, SGPT 310 mU/ml.
Abdominal plain film:	no calcifications in right upper abdomen
Cholescintigraphy I serial scintigraphy (fig. 2-37):	normal visualization of the liver, bile-ducts and gall-bladder. There was no persistent blood-pool activity; excretion of the radiopharmaceutical in the intestine was normal.
Time activity curves: (fig. 2-38)	normal uptake and excretion patterns
Functional images: (fig. 2-39)	normal uptake phase for the right liver lobe, a slightly disturbed uptake phase for the left liver

	lobe and disturbed excretion phase for both liver lobes
Conclusion:	diffuse disturbance of liver parenchyma; left liver lobe more involved than right liver lobe
Liver biopsy:	patterns of hepatitis with cholestatis

Cholescintigraphy was repeated after clinical improvement had set in, but before biochemical liver functions were fully normalized.

Cholescintigraphy II
serial scintigraphy

(fig. 3-40):	an unchanged, normal picture; this was also with the time activity curves
Functional images:	improvement of uptake phase of right liver lobe
(fig. 3-41)	and improvement of excretion phase of both liver lobes.

Case no. 3
A 25-year old male was admitted because of jaundice 2 weeks after taking prescribed medicaments.

Laboratory findings:	total bilirubin 26 umol/l, direct reacting bilirubin 11 μmol/l, alkaline phosphatase 317 mU/ml, SGOT 203 mU/ml, SGPT 439 mU/ml
Abdominal plain film:	no calcifications in the abdomen
Cholescintigraphy	
serial scintigraphy:	good visualization of the liver, there was no
(fig. 4-42)	persistent blood-pool activity; intrahepatic bile-ducts and gall-bladder were visible. Intestinal excretion of the radiopharmaceutical was normal.
Time activity curves:	normal uptake patterns for right and left liver
(fig. 4-43)	lobes. The excretion phase of the right liver lobe is slightly delayed whilst that of the left lobe is normal
Functional images:	normal uptake phase and disturbed excretion phase
(fig. 4-44)	in both liver lobes, in the left lobe more than the right
Conclusion:	no obstruction; suspected of generally disturbed liver parenchyma

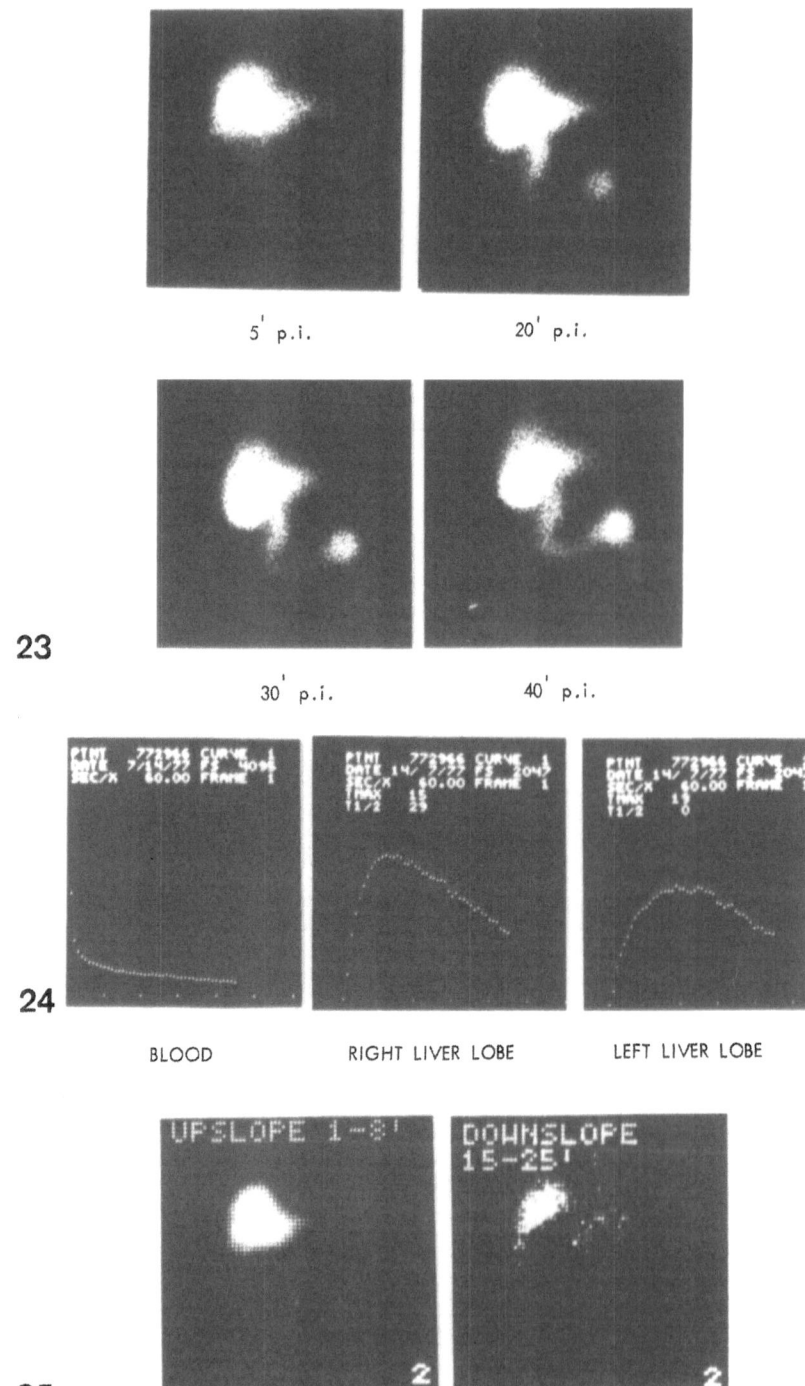

23

5' p.i.   20' p.i.

30' p.i.   40' p.i.

24

BLOOD   RIGHT LIVER LOBE   LEFT LIVER LOBE

25

Fig. 1. 23 - 25: Cholescintigraphy in a patient with cirrhosis in the left liver lobe.

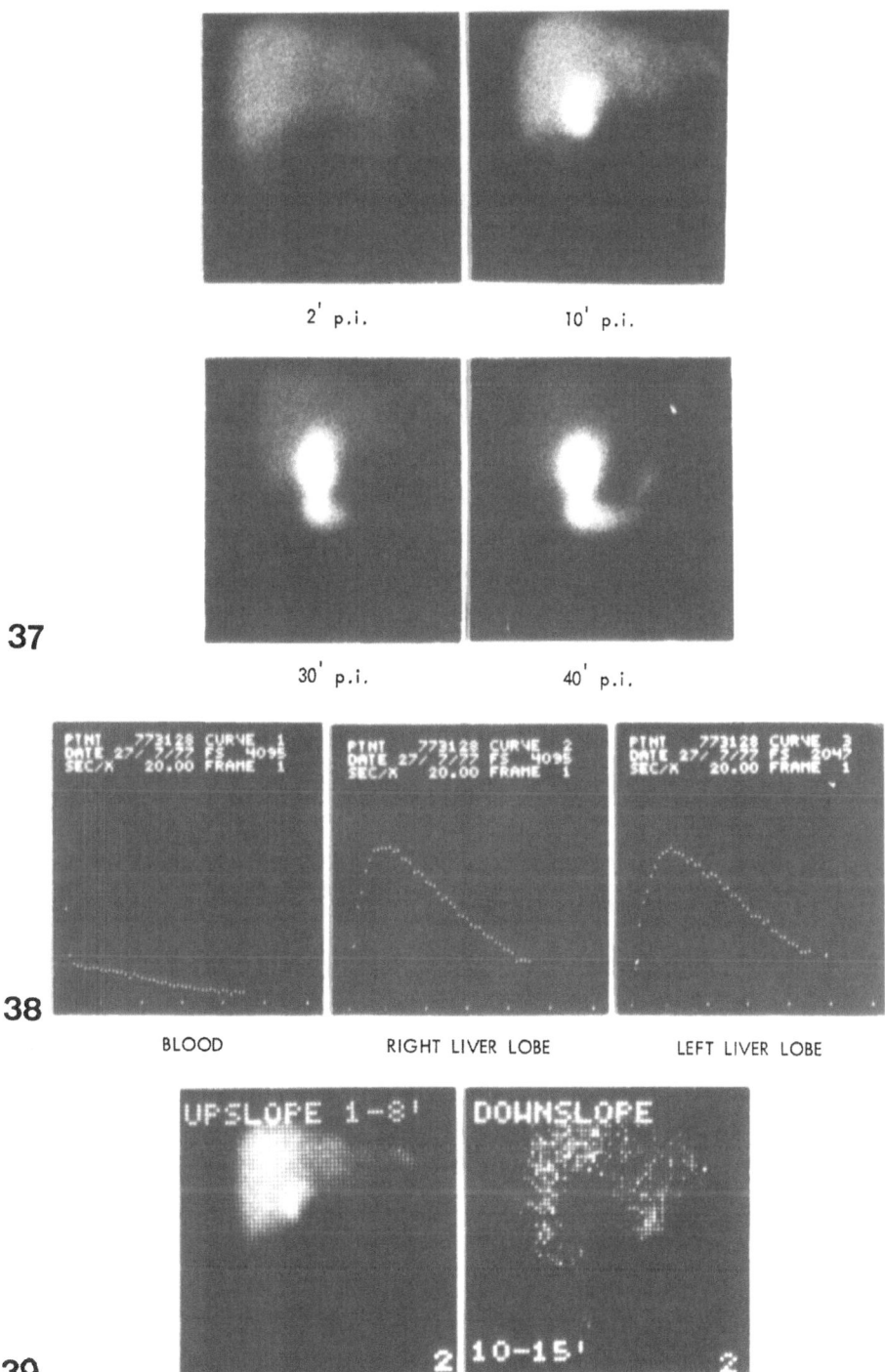

37

2' p.i.   10' p.i.

30' p.i.   40' p.i.

38

BLOOD   RIGHT LIVER LOBE   LEFT LIVER LOBE

39

Fig. 2. 37 - 39: Cholescintigraphy in a patient with probably acute viral hepatitis.

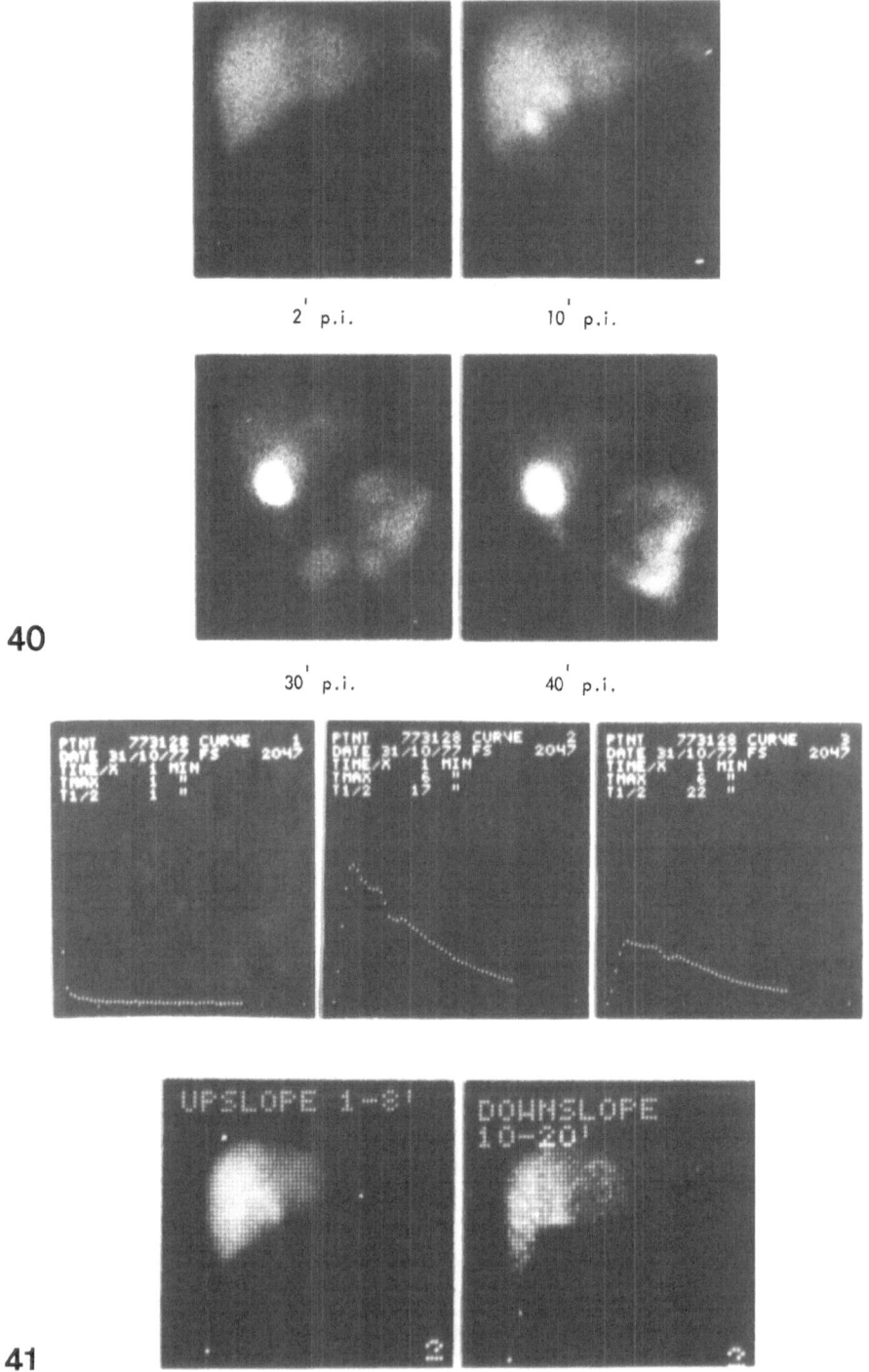

2' p.i.   10' p.i.

30' p.i.   40' p.i.

40

41

Fig. 3. 40 - 41: Cholescintigraphy in a patient with probably acute viral hepatitis; after clinical improvement.

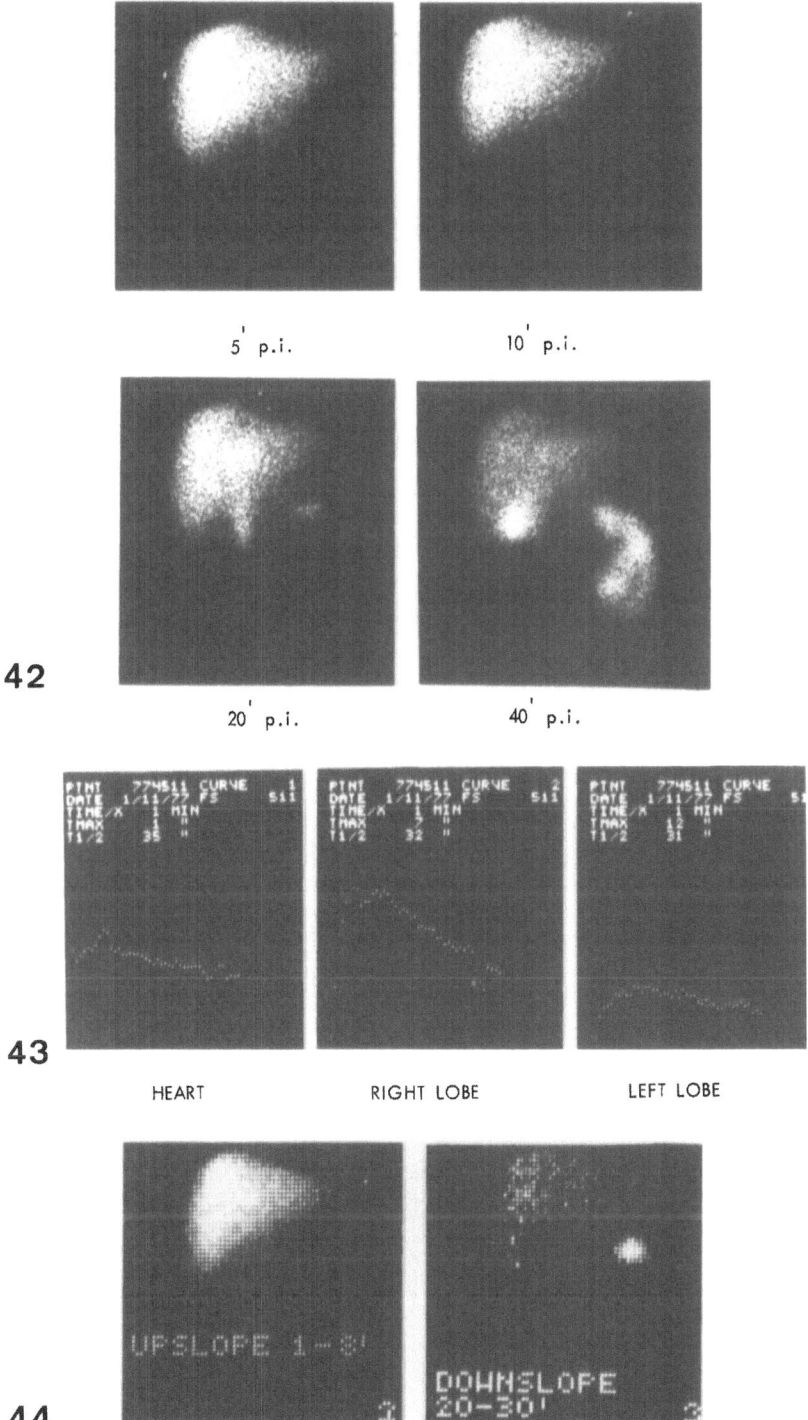

Fig. 4. 42 - 44: Cholescintigraphy in a patient with drug induced hepatitis.

Liver biopsy: patterns that agreed with a diagnosis of drug
                                       induced hepatitis

7.5. Cholescintigraphy in non-jaundiced patients with liver and/or biliary
tract disease

52 patients with various disturbances of liver and biliary tract were investigated. With the exception of 3 patients all patients showed disturbances
in biochemical parameters of liver function, without hyper bilirubinaemia. The
cholescintigraphic investigation was performed routinely to confirm the findings
of other diagnostic investigations and to exclude liver parenchyma disturbance
or aberrations in biliary tract or gall-bladder. The classification of these
patients is shown in table 6.

Table 6. Classification of 52 non-jaundiced patients studied by cholescintigraphy

no. patients	diagnosis
32	parenchymal disease
7	malignant involvement of the liver
10	biliary duct and/or gall-bladder disease
3	various abnormalities

The classification of the patients with liver parenchyma disturbance including
malignant involvement is shown in table 7

Table 7. Classification of 39 non-jaundiced patients with parenchymal liver
disease

no. patients	diagnosis
10	steatosis
1	cirrhosis
4	reactive hepatitis
5	drug induced hepatitis
3	chronic hepatitis
8	aspecific liver function disturbance
7	malignant involvement
1	siderosis

diagnosis	patient no.	alk.phosph. mU/ml	S.G.O.T. mU/ml	S.G.P.T. mU/ml	Y-G.T. mU/ml	intestinal excretion	serial scintigram bile ducts	gallbladder
steatosis	1.	56	36	57	-	N	V	V
hepatis	2.	98	42	71	-	N	V	V
	3.	46	21	52	14	N	V	V
	4.	74	20	17	-	N	V	V
	5.	48	56	54	31	N	V	V
	6.	99	22	55	81	N	V	V
	7.	61	36	51	-	N	V	O
	8.	100	22	19	-	N	V	V
	9.	94	40	39	196	N	V	V
	10.	156	26	63	-	N	V	V
cirrhosis	11.	150	48	44	-	N	V	V
reactive	12.	360	23	48	-	N	V	NV
hepatitis	13.	294	82	103	34	N	NV	V
	14.	116	77	135	28	N	V	V
	15.	174	30	43	-	N	V	V
drug induced	16.	249	71	163	141	N	NV	V
hepatitis	17.	59	178	300	71	N	V	V
	18.	159	23	30	-	N	V	V
	19.	309	29	53	-	N	V	V
	20.	85	152	220	-	N	V	V
chronic	21.	301	25	23	136	N	V	V
hepatitis	22.	154	221	160	-	N	V	NV
	23.	20	17	29	-	N	V	NV
siderosis	24.	104	11	10	-	N	V	V
aspecific	25.	90	19	17	-	N	V	V
liver	26.	96	9	13	-	N	V	O
function	27.	170	13	15	-	N	V	V
disturbance	28.	39	38	43	157	N	V	O
	29.	33	18	19	-	N	V	V
	30.	49	9	4	-	N	V	V
	31.	147	10	8	-	N	V	V
	32.	203	72	30	-	N	NV	V
malignant	33.	500	52	44	-	N	V	V
liver	34.	153	13	11	-	N	NV	NV
involvement	35.	17	13	12	-	N	V	NV
	36.	136	24	30	-	N	V	NV
	37.	112	10	27	-	N	V	V
	38.	34	9	8	-	N	V	V
	39.	149	13	12	-	N	V	V

Table 8. Biochemical blood patterns and findings on the serial scintigram in 39 non-jaundiced patients with parenchymal liver disease, including malignant involvement of the liver.
N= normal. V= visible. NV= non-visible. O= operated.

The final diagnosis was made by liver biopsy, operation or laparoscopy. The 8 patients with aspecific liver function disturbances all showed biochemical aberrations although liver biopsy could not give further information. Table 8 shows the biochemical parameters of the patients studied compared with the findings on the serial scintigram. From the latter intestinal excretion of the radiopharmaceutical and visibility of the bile-duct and gall-bladder are considered. The normal value for alkaline phosphatase is maximal 108 mU/ml, for SGOT 26 mU/ml, for SGPT 26 mU/ml and for gamma glutamyl transpeptidase 4 - 28 mU/ml. As can be seen from table 8 in 10 patients the liver biochemistry was normal. These patients were admitted with disturbed liver function but at the time of cholescintigraphy they were already normalized. Cholescintigraphy was performed to study in how far this investigation could contribute to the diagnosis.

In 9 patients the gall-bladder could not be visualized. In 3 patients (no. 7,26,28) cholecystectomy had been carried out previously. In the other 6 patients, where the gall-bladder could not be visualized, intravenous cholangiography confirmed these findings in 3 cases (no. 22,23,34). In the other 3 no further information about the gall-bladder was obtained, it was possible that these patients were not fasting from 6 hours before the examination. In 1 patient whose gall-bladder could not be visualized laparoscopy showed that it had grown together with the intestines (no. 34). In all of the patients investigated in this series the intestinal excretion of the radiopharmaceutical was normal. In 4 patients there was no clear visualization of the bile-ducts, although in 3 of them the gall-bladder could be seen.

In 38 patients of the patients investigated time activity curves and functional images were generated (table 7). Contrary to the other groups of discussed patients abnormality of the functional images in this series was also viewed for diffuse or focal disturbances.

In 4 patients no aberrations were found either in the time activity curves or in the functional images (no. 4,24,26,31). Patient no. 31 showed a slight evaluation of the alkaline phosphatase level and in the other 3 patients the biochemical blood parameters were normal. In 9 patients was an agreement between the patterns of the time activity curves and the findings in functional imaging. In 6 patients there were normal time activity curves although the downslope functional images for one or both liver lobes were disturbed (no. 1,2,5, 14,35,36). Patient no. 7 showed abnormal downslope images in spite of a normal time activity curve and in addition an abnormal upslope image was also produced

diagnosis	patient no.	T-max right	T-max left	T- liver lobe right	left	Upslope right	left	Downslope right	left	
steatosis	1.	9	9	17	20	N	N	A	A	F
hepatis	2.	11	14	29	26	N	N	A	A	D
	3.	13	15	L	L	N	N	A	A	F
	4.	11	12	24	25	N	N	N	N	
	5.	10	12	22	27	N	N	A	A	F
	6.	9	15	L	17	N	N	A	N	F
	7.	12	13	21	32	N	A	A	A	D
	8.	13	14	27	23	N	A	N	A	F
	9.	13	12	32	33	N	N	A	A	F
	10.	14	23	L	L	N	N	A	A	D
cirrhosis	11.	18	17	L	L	N	N	A	A	D
reactive	12.	9	12	20	33	N	N	A	A	F
hepatitis	13.	-	-	-	-	-	-	-	-	-
	14.	9	9	19	18	N	N	N	A	F
	15.	14	14	20	L	N	N	A	A	D
drug induced	16.	10	11	34	32	N	N	A	A	D
hepatitis	17.	13	19	22	L	N	N	A	A	F
	18.	13	10	L	34	N	N	A	A	D
	19.	22	36	L	L	N	N	N	A	F
	20.	15	13	L	L	N	N	A	A	D
chronic	21.	14	15	L	L	N	N	A	A	D
hepatitis	22.	23	14	L	L	N	N	A	A	D
	23.	23	33	L	L	N	N	A	A	F
siderosis	24.	3	10	19	17	N	N	N	N	
aspecific	25.	14	15	L	L	N	N	A	A	F
liver	26.	6	11	27	24	N	N	N	N	
function	27.	15	19	23	35	N	N	A	A	D
disturbance	28.	16	13	L	17	N	N	A	N	F
	29.	15	14	L	29	N	N	A	A	D
	30.	19	AC	27	AC	A	A	A	A	D
	31.	12	11	22	23	N	N	N	N	
	32.	30	33	L	L	N	N	A	A	D
malignant	33.	AC	AC	AC	AC	N	A	A	A	D
liver	34.	15	18	30	L	N	N	A	A	F D
involvement	35.	9	8	23	22	N	N	N	A	F
	36.	3	10	27	30	N	N	A	A	D
	37.	21	AC	L	A	N	N	A	A	F
	38.	14	26	31	L	N	N	A	A	F
	39.	4	32	L	L	N	N	A	A	F

Table 9. Computer data of 39 non-jaundiced patients with parenchymal liver disease, including malignant involvement of the liver.
AC= ascending curve. L= lengthened. N= normal. A= abnormal. F= focal. D= diffuse.
T max and $T\frac{1}{2}$ are in minutes.

in spite of a normal maximum uptake time for the left liver lobe; the patient was suffering from an extensive steatosis of the liver.

3 Patients had disturbed downslope images in spite of normal half value time of the curves, however in these patients the maximum uptake time for the liver was delayed (no. 15,27,30). In 2 of these patients (no. 15,27) the upslope image was normal although the maximum uptake time was slightly delayed. This latter finding was also seen in 14 other patients in whom the time activity curve implied a delayed uptake of the reagent by the liver; the upslope functional image however was normal.

One patient with failure to visualize the gall-bladder in oral cholecystography was suffering from liver cirrhosis (table 9 no.11). IVC could not be

Table 10. Diagnostic investigation in 39 non-jaundiced patients with liver parenchymal disturbance

diagnostic investigation	no. patients	visualization of liver and/or biliary tract	
		success	failure
percutaneous liver biopsy	27	27	-
colloid liver scintigraphy	25	25	-
abdominal plain film	6	-	-
oral cholecystography	12	9	3
intravenous cholangio-graphy	10	7	3
ultrasound study	4	4	-
arteriography	1	1	-
laparoscopy	3	3	-

performed in this patient because he was allergic for intravenously administered contrast material. 2 patients with non-visualization of the gall-bladder on oral cholecystography also showed no gall-bladder on intravenous cholangiography (no. 23,24). The non-visualization of the gall-bladder could not be confirmed by surgery. Intravenous cholangiography showed in 1 patient, suffering from aspecific liver function disturbance (no. 28), excretion of the contrast material by the kidneys and a very poor visualization of the bile-ducts. Table 11 compares the results of cholescintigraphy and the results of some investigations in diagnosing a parenchymal disturbance of the liver. Colloid liver scintigram was performed in 25 patients. In 16 patients the scintigraphic findings were suspected for pathology of the liver i.e. enlarged liver, inhomogeneous distribution of the radiocolloid and/or space occupying processes. In 1 patient a lesion in the right liver lobe was suspected; this could not be confirmed.

Percutaneous liver biopsy showed no abnormalities in 2 patients: 1 patient was suffering from reactive hepatitis, another has multiple metastases in the liver. In 5 patients liver biopsy showed atypical pattern; no diagnosis could be made on the specimen obtained (table 11 between brackets). Ultrasound showed no aberrations in 3 patients suffering respectively from steatosis, chronic hepatitis and metastases. In 1 patient an ultrasound study was positive for multiple cystic processes but surgery showed multiple solid metastases in the liver. Cholescintigraphy showed no aberrations in 4 patient, either in the serial scintigram or in time activity curves or functional images. In all other patients there was a disturbed downslope phase in functional images in spite of a normal intestinal excretion of the reagent on the serial scintigram. Time activity curves were normal in 7 patients in whom functional imaging showed a disturbed excretion phase.

Table 11. Frequency of correct diagnosing of investigations in non-jaundiced patients with parenchymal liver disease

diagnostic investigation	no. patients	no abnormalities	correct diagnosis	other diagnosis
percutaneous liver biopsy	27	2 (5)	20	-
colloid liver scintigraphy	25	9	15	1
ultrasound study	4	3	-	1
laparoscopy	3	2	1	-
cholescinti- graphy	38	4	34	-

7.6. Discussion

The results of the study revealed the following patterns of cholescintigraphy in patients with biochemical indications of liver function disturbance without jaundice.

Serial scintigraphy. All patients showed normal intestinal excretion. No persistent blood-pool activity was observed. Bile-ducts were visible in 90% of the patients studied. In 86% of the patients with malignant involvement of the liver the serial scintigram showed no abnormalities. In 14% space occupying processes were observed.

Time activity curves:

34% of the patients studied showed normal maximum uptake time and normal half value time for both liver lobes.

- normal T max for both liver lobes was observed in 47% of the patients studied
- delayed T max for both liver lobes was observed in 24%
- delayed T max for only the right liver lobe was observed in 16%
- delayed T max for only the left lobe was observed in 5%
- ascending curve for both liver lobes was observed in 3%
- ascending curve for left liver lobe and delayed T max for right lobe was observed in 5%
- normal T½ for both liver lobes was observed in 34% of the patient studied
- lengthened T½ for both liver lobes was observed in 34%
- lengthened T½ for only the right lobe was observed in 11%
- lengthened T½ for only the left lobe was observed in 13%
- ascending curve for both liver lobes was observed in 3%
- ascending curve for left liver lobe was observed in 5%

Functional imaging:

- the upslope and downslope images were normal for both liver lobes in 10%
- the upslope and downslope images were abnormal for both liver lobes in 3%
- the upslope images normal, downslope images abnormal for both liver lobes in 66%
- the downslope images was abnormal for one of the liver lobes when other functional images were normal in 13%
- the upslope image was normal for the right liver lobe whilst other images were abnormal in 5%
- the upslope and downslope image of the right lobe were normal whilst upslope and downslope image of the left lobe were abnormal in 3%

7.7. Clinical reliability

All patients in this study showed a normal intestinal excretion on the serial scintigram; diagnosis parenchymal liver disease on the serial scintigram only was possible in this study. The computer data showed an indication of bile-duct obstruction in 8% of the patients studied whilst no liver function distur-bance was indicated in 10% of the patients studied. The success rate for the computer data in diagnosing liver parenchyma disturbance was therefore 82%. In comparison the success rate in diagnosing parenchymal disease was for percutaneous liver biopsy 74%, for colloid liver-scintigraphy 60%, for laparoscopy 33%. Ultrasound could not diagnose parenchymal disease in the patients studied.

7.8. Case histories

Let us conclude by studying several case histories in detail to illustrate this group of patients.

Case no. 4

A 45-year old female was admitted because of slight biochemical liver function disturbance and an enlarged liver. There was a prior history of alcohol abuse.

Laboratory findings:	total bilirubin 15 umol/l, direct reacting bilirubin 2 μmol/l, alkaline phosphatase 136 mU/ml, SGOT 42 mU/ml, SGPT 24 mU/ml
Colloid liverscintigraphy:	enlarged liver with inhomogeneous activity distribution; space occupying processes could not be excluded
Cholescintigraphy serial scintigram: (fig. 5-1)	enlarged liver, visibility of intrahepatic bile-ducts and gall-bladder, inhomogeneous distribution of the radiopharmaceutical. Normal intestinal excretion of the reagent.
Time activity curves: (fig. 5-2)	normal uptake and excretion patterns
Functional images: (fig. 5-3)	disturbed uptake left liver lobe, slight disturbed excretion phase right liver lobe, strongly disturbed excretion left liver lobe
Conclusion:	suspicion of liver parenchyma disturbance
Liver biopsy:	alcoholic hepatitis and steatosis

Case no. 5

A 56-year old male was admitted because of enlarged liver and disturbed liver biochemistry.

Laboratory findings:	total bilirubin 13 umol/l, direct reacting bilirubin 2 μmol/l, alkaline phosphatase 301 mU/ml, SGOT 25 mU/ml, SGPT 23 mU/ml, gamma GT 136 mU/ml

112

Colloid liverscintigraphy:	enlarged liver, no further aberrations

Cholescintigraphy

serial scintigram: (fig. 6-4)	good visualization of the liver, gall-bladder and bile-ducts. Normal intestinal excretion of the reagent
Time activity curves: (fig. 6-5)	slightly delayed maximum uptake time in the right liver lobe, normal maximum uptake time in left liver lobe, lengthened half value time in both liver lobes
Functional images: (fig. 6-6)	upslope image showed normal uptake phase, down-slope image showed diffuse disturbed excretion phase
Conclusion:	suspicion of diffuse liver parenchyma disturbance
Liver biopsy:	chronic active hepatitis

Case no. 6

A 58-year old female was admitted because of disturbed liver biochemistry.

Laboratory findings:	total bilirubin 13 μmol/l, direct reacting bilirubin 2 μmol/l, alkaline phosphatase 85 mU/ml, SGOT 152 mU/ml, SGPT 220 mU/ml

Cholescintigraphy

serial scintigram: (fig. 7-7)	good visualization of the liver, bile-ducts and gall-bladder. Normal intestinal excretion of the radiopharmaceutical
Time activity curves: (fig. 7-8)	normal maximum uptake time for both liver lobes, lengthened half value time for both liver lobes
Functional images: (fig. 7-9)	upslope image shows normal uptake phase, down-slope image showes general disturbed excretion phase
Conclusion:	suspect for liver parenchyma disturbance
Liver biopsy:	patterns suspect for a drug induced hepatitis

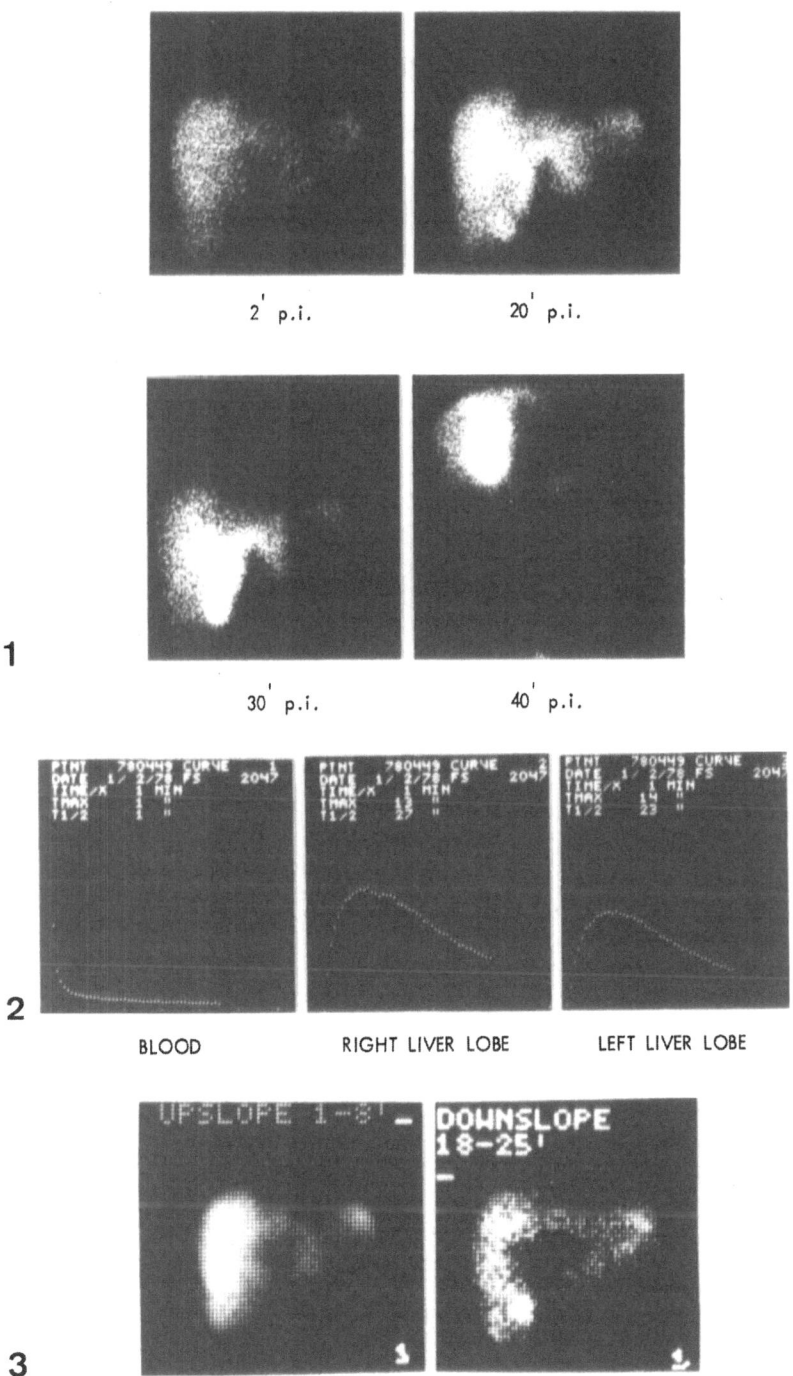

Fig. 5. 1 - 3: Cholescintigraphy in a patient with alcoholic hepatitis and steatosis.

114

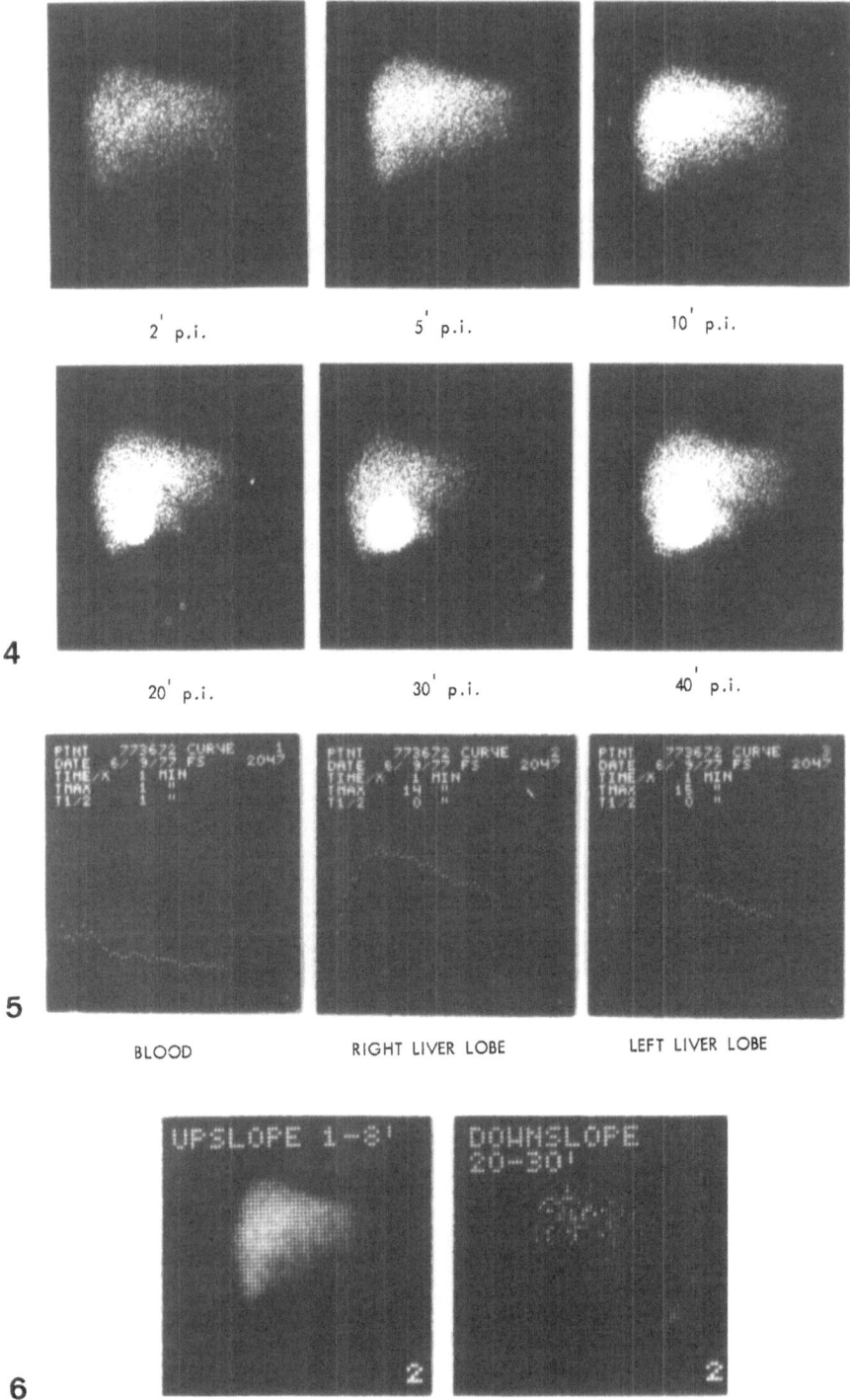

Fig. 6. 4 - 6: Cholescintigraphy in a patient with chronic active hepatitis.

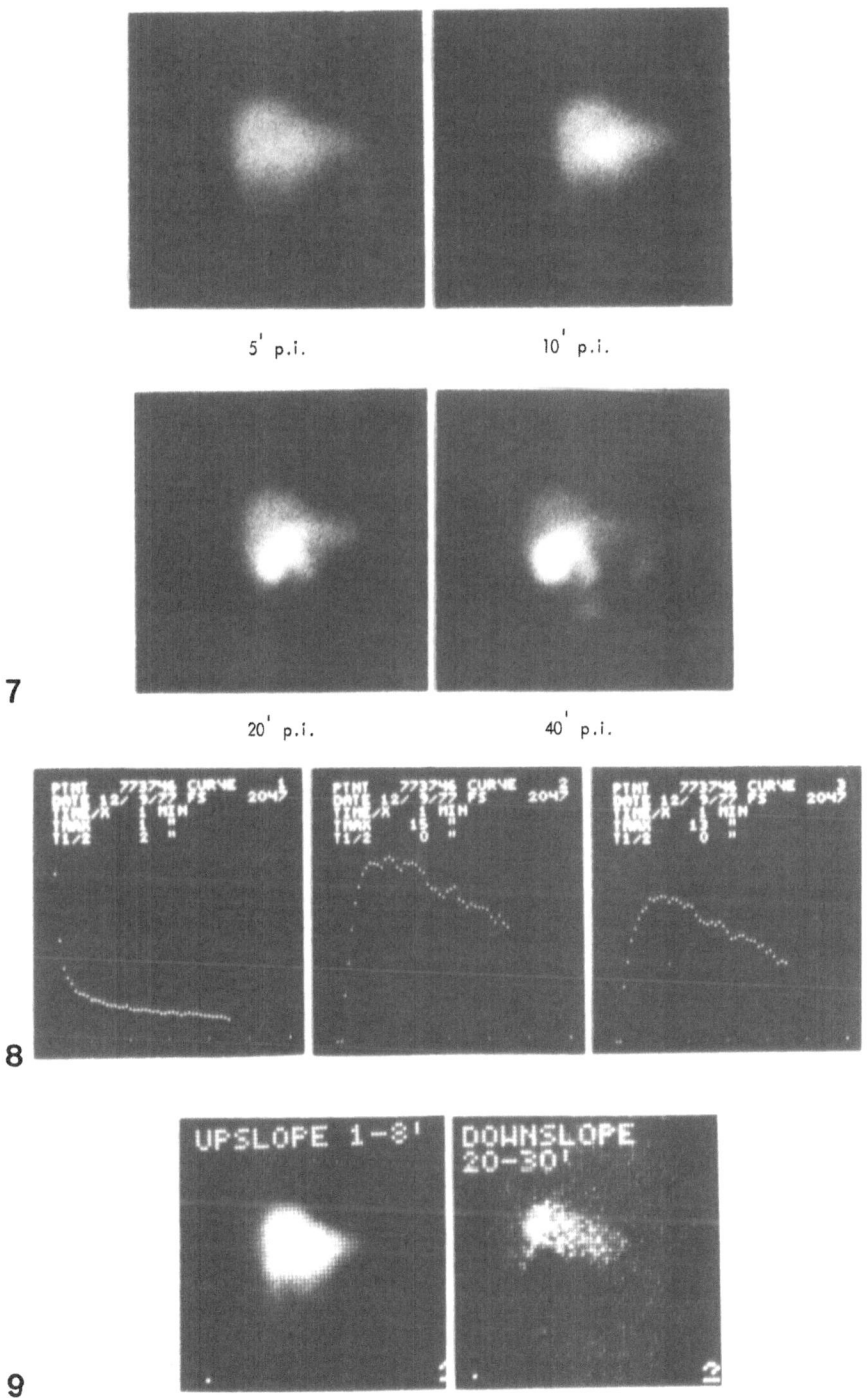

5' p.i.   10' p.i.

7

20' p.i.   40' p.i.

8

9

Fig. 7. 7 - 9: Cholescintigraphy in a patient with a drug induced hepatitis.

REFERENCES

1. Tjen HSLM, Cholescintigraphy Ph.D. Thesis, University of Utrecht, The Netherlands (in English), 1979.

2. Biersack HJ, Mahlstedt J, Hepatobiliäre Funktionsszintigraphie mit Ida-Derivaten. Proceedings of the symposium North-Rine Westpahalian Society of Nuclear Medicine,1978. Biersack HJ, Mahlstedt J (eds), Darmstadt, G-I-T/E Giebler, 1978.

3. Cox PH, Progress in Radiopharmacology, Vol.I. Cox PH (ed), Amsterdam, Elsevier/North-Holland Biomedical Press, 1979.

4. NucComp 3:66, 1978.

8. CHOLESCINTIGRAPHY IN OBSTRUCTIVE DISEASE

H.S.L.M. TJEN, P.H. COX

8.I. INTRODUCTION

Cholescintigraphy has proved to be a useful tool in evaluating obstructive liver disease (1,2,3,4) even in patients with very high bilirubin levels. Diethyl-Ida has until now been the reagent most widely used but it has been suggested (5) that quantitative studies are necessary for optimal diagnosis.

Parabutyl-Ida with its lower urinary excretion level even at high serum bilirubin levels appears to give a better liver visualization in extreme cases but its slow liver turnover even in normal subjects can give confusing results and may lead to misinterpretation of scintigrams especially in follow-up (6).

In our Institute (7) in 1978 a study of 45 patients with obstructive disease of the biliary tract was made. They could be differentiated into 22 patients with obstruction from a tumour in the head of the pancreas, 7 patients with an obstructing tumour in the liver-hilus and 16 patients with an obstruction in the common bile-duct to stones and/or inflammation. All diagnoses were confirmed by operation or post mortem investigation. In table 1 the findings on the serial scintigrams prepared using Diethyl-Ida are shown.

8.2. Results in patients with pancreas head tumour

22 patients with a proven tumour in pancreas head were investigated in this study. All showed progressive jaundice, raised alkaline phosphatase and slight to moderate elevation of serum transaminases. Cholescintigraphy using serial scintigrams showed complete obstruction in 20 patients (91.3%). In 2 patients there was delayed intestinal excretion, due to partial obstruction. These 2 patients had relatively low bilirubin values: 103 and 114 µmol/l whilst the alkaline phosphatase activity was 1500 and 177 mU/ml respectively.

The serial scintigrams of patients with complete obstruction showed 2 types of pattern. In 10 patients there was a moderate persistence of blood-pool activity and a relative good visualization of the liver. Neither bile-duct nor intestinal activity could be observed 24 hours post injection. In the other

118

Table 1. Frequency of organ visualization in 45 obstructive patients

diagnosis	no. patients	liver	visualization of gall-bladder	bile-ducts	intestine
pancreas head tumour	22	10	0	0	2
liver hilus tumour	7	4	0	0	2
stones in common bile-duct	7	6	0	4	6
cholangitis	2	2	0	0	2
stones in common bile-duct and gall-bladder	7	7	0	4	5

10 patients with complete obstruction there was a poor visualization of the liver associated with persistent high blood-pool activity. In some cases the liver could hardly be distinguished from blood-pool. In 16 patients of the 20 patients with complete obstruction, excretion of the reagent by the kidneys was observed. There was no correlation between bilirubin values and the observed scintigraphic patterns in these patients. In the first mentioned type of serial scintigrams bilirubin ranges varying from 100 to 360 µmol/l in the latter the range varied from 198 - 624 µmol/l.

Time activity curves and functional images were generated from the data stored in the computer. As routine the one minute frames during the first 8 to 10 minutes of the study were compressed to produce a cumulative image. In this way a clearer image of both the liver and intrahepatic structures was obtained. In this series it was only possible to generate the curves and functional images from 8 patients in whom a relative good visualization of the liver on the serial scintigram was obtained.

In all other cases the uptake of the radiopharmaceutical in the liver was so poor that only curves and functional images of blood-pool were obtained. In table 2 the values for maximum uptake time (T max) and half value time for excretion ($T\frac{1}{2}$) are shown in comparison with the functional images, bilirubin values and serial scintigrams. The maximum uptake times for right and left liver lobes are prolonged whilst the half value time for the excretion phase was not calculated because it exceeded the total time of the examination.

The excretion phase shows 3 characteristic curves:

1. half value time is prolonged (L),
2. the curve develops into a plateau after a maximum uptake value is reached (P),
3. there is a continously ascending curve during the whole period of the study (AC).

The 2 patients whose curves show a plateau for both liver lobes were confirmed as patients with complete obstruction due to a pancreas head tumour with liver metastases. The patient with continously ascending curve proved to have a complete obstruction due to a pancreas head tumour. Both patients with a prolonged half value time for both liver lobes, showed complete obstruction in the serial scintigram, however in one of these patients this could not be confirmed by surgery. The functional images in all the 8 patients show a normal upslope, demonstrating that the hepatocyte uptake of the radiopharmaceutical is normal although uptake was somewhat delayed in some cases, as can be seen on the time activity curves. In 6 patients the downslope was considered to be abnormal demonstrating that the hepatocyte is able to excrete although the excretion phase is disturbed.

Table 2. Maximum uptake time and half value time of the time activity curves of 8 patients with pancreas head tumour in comparison with functional imaging, bilirubin values and intestinal excretion on serial scintigram.

C= complete obstruction. D= delayed excretion. L= lengthened. P= plateau. AC= ascending curve. N= normal. A= abnormal. BPA= blood-pool activity. T max and $T\frac{1}{2}$ are in minutes. Right= right liver lobe. Left= left liver lobe.

total bilirubin μmol/l	intestinal excretion serial scintigram	T max		$T\frac{1}{2}$		upslope		downslope	
		right	left	right	left	right	left	right	left
198	C	19	18	L	L	N	N	A	A
110	C	20	30	L	P	N	N	A	A
103	D	10	14	L	P	N	N	A	A
114	D	30	26	P	L	N	N	A	A
372	C	17	23	P	P	N	N	BPA	BPA
200	C	10	14	L	L	N	N	A	A
280	C	14	21	P	P	N	N	A	A
173	C	AC	AC	AC	AC	N	N	BPA	BPA

In the investigation of the patients with a finally confirmed extrahepatic
obstruction due to pancreas head tumour the following examinations were initial-
ly performed to determine whether the jaundice had an extrahepatic or an intrahepatic cause. See table 3.

Table 3. Clinical investigation in 22 patients with bile-duct obstruction by
tumour in pancreas head

diagnostic investigation	no. patients	visualization of liver and/or bile-ducts	
		success	failure
abdominal plain film	9	-	-
oral cholecystography	1	0	1
arteriography	1	1	0
percutaneous trans-hepatic cholangio-graphy	10	9	1
ultrasound study	12	12	0
colloid liverscinti-graphy	11	11	0

In 3 patients abdominal plain film showed calcifications in the right upper
abdomen; in none of these patients were stones found in gall-bladder or bile-
ducts. In the other 6 patients no further information could be obtained with
this examination. The oral cholecystography was performed in a patient with a
total bilirubin of 200 μmol/l. Arteriography of coeliac trunk and superior
mesenteric artery did not demonstrate pathology. In 3 patients the colloid
scintigram of the liver indicated the presence of space occupying lesion, which
was confirmed in all cases by surgery, 1 patient showed a normal liver scintigram, 1 patient diminished activity in liver hilus and 6 patients an atypical
inhomogeneous distribution of radioactivity in the liver. The success rate in
diagnosing extrahepatic obstruction of percutaneous transhepatic cholangiography (PTC) and ultrasound study is given in table 4 and compared with the
results of cholescintigraphy.

Criteria for the diagnosis of extrahepatic obstruction are the dilated bile-
ducts on the image obtained by PTC and ultrasound and for cholescintigraphy the
delay or absence of excretion on the serial scintigram, eventually combined with
typical patterns obtained from the computer. 1 patient showed a slight flow of
contrast to the duodenum in the PTC study though the serial scintigram showed a

Table 4. Frequency of visualization of obstruction patterns in PTC ultrasound and cholescintigraphy

	no. patients	dilated bile-ducts	dilated gall-bladder	intestinal excretion	correct diagnosis
percutaneous transhepatic cholangiography	9	8	3	1	8
ultrasound study	12	9	6		9
cholescintigraphy	22			2	22

complete obstruction. Time activity curves from this patient show a normal up-take and delayed excretion of the radiopharmaceutical by the liver; the function-al images show a normal upslope and slightly disturbed downslope. With regard to these findings there is also an agreement with the findings on the PTC and the condition observed at operation.

The delayed excretion on the serial scintigrams in 2 patients was inter-preted as due to partial obstruction, because the time activity curves showed a plateau after the maximum uptake time was reached in at least one of the liver lobes. PTC was performed in one of these patients; no contrast flow into duodenum was seen. Similarly the findings of the ultrasound did not agree with the findings by operation. It should be mentioned that only in 3 patients the ultrasound study was suspect for the pathology of the pancreas; in 3 patients there was a suspicion of stones in the gall-bladder, though in none of these patients gall-bladder stones were found. In 1 patient with multiple stones in the gall-bladder, no stones were found with ultrasound.

The results of this study revealed the following patterns of cholescinti-graphy in patients with an obstructive jaundice due to pancreas head tumour.

Serial scintigraphy:
- abnormal intestinal excretion was always observed
- delayed intestinal excretion was observed in 8./% of the patients studied
- complete obstruction was observed in 91.3% of the patients studied.

Patients with a complete obstruction showed:
- good liver visualization with persistence of a slight blood-pool activity in 50% of the cases studied
- poor liver visualization with persistence of a high level of blood-pool activ-ity in the other 50%.

Patients with delayed intestinal excretion all showed:
- good liver visualisation with a slight persistence of blood-pool activity.

Computer data: No additional information could be obtained with the
computer in 64% of the patients studied. Time activity curves obtained from the
patients with a complete obstruction showed the following patterns:
- normal T max for both liver lobes in 17% of the patients studied
- delayed T max for both liver lobes in 66%
- a lengthened $T\frac{1}{2}$ for both liver lobes was observed in 33% of the patients
  studied
- in both liver lobes the curve showed a plateau after T max has been reached
  in 33% of the patients studied while in a further 17% only the left lobe was
  so affected
- continuously ascending curve for both liver lobes in 17% of the patients
  studied.

Time activity curves for the patients with a delayed excretion showed the
following patterns:
- normal T max for both liver lobes in 50%
- delayed T max for both liver lobes in 50%
- the time activity curve showed a plateau in 50% for the right lobe and in
  50% for the left lobe.

Functional images obtained from all patients studied showed the following
patterns:
- upslope image revealed a normal uptake phase in 100% of the patients studied
- downslope images revealed a disturbed phase in 100% of the patients studied.

Clinical reliability: Extrahepatic obstruction could be surmized if there
was a complete obstruction on the serial scintigram. In this series of patients
extrahepatic obstruction was indicated on the serial scintigram in 91.3% of the
cases. Extrahepatic obstruction was indicated by the computer data when the
time activity curves of one or both liver lobes either developed a plateau after
the maximum uptake was reached or showed a continuous increase during the whole
study. When serial scintigram patterns were combined with the results of the
computer analysis the overall success rate for cholescintigraphy is diagnosing
extrahepatic obstruction in these patients was 100%. In this group percutaneous
transhepatic cholangiography showed a success rate of 88% In diagnosing extrahepatic obstruction, whilst the success rate for ultrasound study was 75%. A
typical case history is given by the following example:

A 75-years old male was admitted because of persistent pain in the right
upper abdomen of more than 6 weeks duration and associated with persistent
jaundice. On physical examination a slightly jaundiced man with an enlarged

liver was presented.

Laboratory findings:	total bilirubin 110 μmol/l, direct reacting bilirubin 83 μmol/l, alkaline phosphatase 410 mU/ml, SGOT 320 mU/ml, SGPT 700 mU/ml
colloid liver scintigraphy:	diminished activity in liver hilus
ultrasound:	enlarged bile-ducts in liver hilus
percutaneous transhepatic cholangiography:	distended common bile-duct, no entrance of contrast in duodenum
cholescintigraphy serial scintigraphy:	good visualization of the liver, no visible bile-ducts or gall-bladder. No intestinal activity 24 hours post injection
cumulative picture: (fig. 1-3)	"cold" area in liver hilus
time activity curves: (fig. 1-4)	maximum uptake time for both right and left lobes is delayed. The curve from right liver lobe shows a very prolonged excretion, the curve from left liver lobe shows a plateau
functional images: (fig. 1-5)	upslope shows no aberration, the downslope functional image is diffusely disturbed
conclusion:	suspected bile-duct obstruction
operative findings:	distended common bile-duct; peroperative cholangiography showed no passage of contrast material into duodenum. Stenosis of common bile-duct by adenocarcinoma of the head of the pancreas.

8.3. Results in patients with tumour in liver hilus

7 patients with progressive jaundice due to an obstruction of the bile-ducts in liver hilus were investigated. The cholescintigraphic investigation showed in 5 patients (71%) a complete obstruction on the serial scintigram and in 2 patients (29%) a delayed intestinal excretion due to partial obstruction of the bile-ducts. In these latter patients the bilirubin values were 170 μmol/l and 210 μmol/l and the alkaline phosphatase values were respectively 928 mU/ml and 55 mU/ml. As in the case of patients with a pancreas head tumour the patterns of the serial scintigrams in the completely obstructed patients are similar and

124

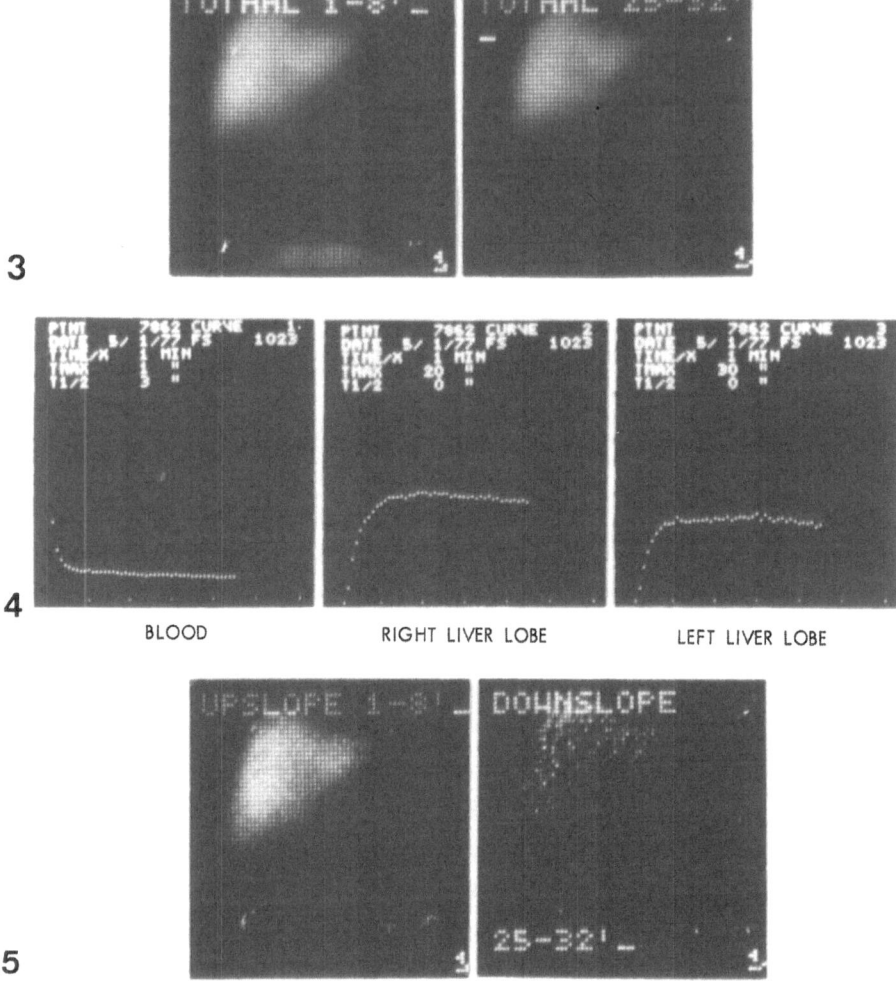

3

4

BLOOD   RIGHT LIVER LOBE   LEFT LIVER LOBE

5

and are distinguished in "good" liver visualization and "bad" liver visualization. Also no relation between the type of pattern observed and bilirubin
value was seen. In all of these patients cumulative images, time activity
curves and functional images were generated from the computer data. The cumulative images more clearly demonstrated a pathological process in the liver-
hilus in 4 patients where this was suspected from the images of the serial scintigram. In table 5 the values for maximum uptake time and half value time for
the excretory phase are shown, in comparison with the functional images, bilirubin values and intestinal excretion.

Table 5. Maximum uptake time and half value time of the time activity curves of
7 patients with bile-duct obstruction in liver hilus in comparison with funtion-
al images, bilirubin values and excretion on serial scintigram.

C= complete obstruction. D= delayed excretion. L= lengthened. P= plateau. BPA=
blood-pool activity. N= normal. Λ= abnormal.

total bilirubin μmol/l	intestinal excretion	T max right left		T½ right left		upslope right left		downslope right left	
400	C	BPA		BPA		BPA		BPA	
173	C	20	18	L	L	N	N	A	A
150	C	18	30	P	P	N	N	A	A
655	C	BPA		BPA		BPA		BPA	
170	D	16	16	L	L	N	N	A	A
150	C	BPA		BPA		BPA		BPA	
210	D	18	19	L	P	N	N	A	A

In 3 patients the time activity curves and functional images could not be
generated because no uptake of the radiopharmaceutical by the liver was observed. In 2 patients there were diffuse metastases in the liver; in 1 patient
there was a massive space occupying lesion in the left liver lobe originating
from the hilus of a much congested liver. In 1 patient, showing a delayed excretion, there was an almost normal maximum uptake time and prolonged half
value time. In the 3 other patients the maximum uptake time was slightly delayed. Of these 3 patients, 2 showed lengthened half value time for the excretion
phase instead of a plateau, though complete obstruction was proven. Table 6
shows the other clinical investigation in these patients compared with the
frequency of visualization of liver and/or bile-ducts.

Table 6. Clinical investigation in 7 patients with bile-duct obstruction by tumour in liver hilus. Frequency of visualization of liver and/or bile-ducts

diagnostic investigation	no. patients	visualization of liver and/or bile ducts	
		success	failure
abdominal plain film	2	-	-
oral cholecystography	1	0	1
intravenous cholangiography	2	0	2
percutaneous trans-hepatic cholangio-graphy	3	3	0
ultrasound study	4	4	0
colloid liver scintigraphy	5	5	0

1 patient who underwend a PTC developed complications due to bile leakage and peritonitis. The patients in whom oral and intravenous cholangiography failed, had bilirubin values of 150 - 173 μmol/l. In table 7 the frequency of occurence of obstruction patterns as dilated bile-ducts and/or stenosis in liver hilus and the success rate of diagnosing extrahepatic obstruction by these investigations is shown.

Table 7. Frequency of visualization of obstruction patterns and success rate in diagnozing extrahepatic obstruction in PTC, ultrasound and cholescintigraphy

diagnostic investigation	no. patients	dilated bile-ducts	stenosis liver hilus	intestinal excretion	correct diagnosis
percutaneous transhepatic cholangiography	3	2	3		3
ultrasound study	4	2			2
cholescintigraphy	7			2	7

The findings on the serial scintigram in regard to intestinal excretion could not be confirmed in these patients by other investigations. All operated patients showed an obstructing, malignant tumour in the liver hilus; in none of these patients however was an attempt made to check whether the obstruction was total or sub-total. In the 2 patients with delayed excretion no confirmation of partial bile-duct obstruction could be obtained from PTC. A correct diagnosis for PTC was recorded if this investigation was able to show dilated intrahepatic bile-ducts and the site of obstruction. Ultrasound showed dilated bile-ducts in only 2 patients but gave no information as to the site and extension of the obstruction.

Liverscintigraphy was performed in 5 patients; in 3 patients there was a suspicion of a process in the liver hilus. A correct diagnosis for cholescintigraphy was recorded if this investigation was able to show extrahepatic obstruction. In 5 patients extrahepatic obstruction was suspected because a complete obstruction on the serial scintigram could be seen. In 1 patient extrahepatic obstruction was suspected because of delayed excretion on the serial scintigram and a time activity curve from the left liver lobe which showed a plateau for the excreting phase. In the other patient with delayed intestinal excretion and lengthened half value time of the time activity curves from both liver lobes, which signs could be also suspect for a diffuse lever parenchyma disturbance, the serial scintigram and cumulative images showed a persistent cold area in liver hilus. This finding was therefore suspect for an obstructing process in liver hilus.

The results of the study in patients with obstructive jaundice due to a malignant tumour in liver hilus showed the following patterns of cholescintigraphy.

Serial scintigraphy:
- no cases with normal intestinal excretion patterns were observed
- delayed excretion was observed in 29% of the patients studied
- suspicion of a pathological process in liver hilus was observed in 67%.
Patients with a complete obstruction showed:
- good liver visualization with persistence of a slight blood-pool activity in 40% of the cases
- poor liver visualization with persistence of a high blood-pool activity in 60%.
Patients with delayed intestinal excretion all showed:
- a good liver visualization with persistence of a slight blood-pool activity.

Computer data: No additional information from the computer analysis was obtained in 43% of the patients studied. Time activity curves obtained from patients with a complete obstruction showed the following patterns:
- delayed T max for both liver lobes in all cases
- lengthened $T\frac{1}{2}$ for both liver lobes in 50%

- a plateau following the T max for both liver lobes in 50%.

Time activity curves obtained from the patients with a delayed intestinal excretion showed the following patterns:

- normal T max for both liver lobes in one of the patients

- delayed T max for both liver lobes in another patient

- lengthenes $T\frac{1}{2}$ for both liver lobes in 1 patient

- the curve revealed a plateau for the left liver lobe in another patient.

Functional images obtained from all the patients studied showed the following patterns:

- upslope image revealed a normal uptake phase in 100% of the patients studied

- downslope image revealed a disturbed excretion phase in 100% of the patients studied.

Clinical reliability: Extrahepatic obstruction could be diagnosed on the serial scintigram when there was a complete obstruction. In this series of patients extrahepatic obstruction could be diagnosed on the basis of the serial scintigram alone in 71%. The possibility of extrahepatic obstruction was also present if a persistent cold area in the liver hilus could be observed on the serial scintigram without complete obstruction being present. In relation to this latter pattern when combined with the results where complete obstruction was observed on the serial scintigram extrahepatic obstruction was diagnosed in 86% of the cases studied.

The computer results indicated extrahepatic obstruction when there was a cold area in the liver hilus on the cumulative image, when time activity curves showed a plateau after reaching maximum uptake time for one or both liver lobes or when the curve continued ascending during the whole study. When serial scintigram patterns were combined with computer data the overall success rate for cholescintigraphy in diagnosing extrahepatic obstruction in patients with obstructive jaundice due to a liver hilus tumour was 100%. The success rate in this study for percutaneous transhepatic cholangiography was 100% and for ultrasound study 50% in diagnosing extrahepatic obstruction.

8.4. Results in patients with non-malignant obstruction of the common bile-duct

16 jaundiced patients with a non-malignant obstruction of the common bile-duct were investigated. The classification of these patients according to the diagnosis is shown in table 8. Of the patients with common bile-duct stones in 6 cases gall-bladder stones were also found at operation; 2 patients had a cholecystectomy at an ealier date. The diagnosis of the patient with the

perforation of the gall-bladder was obtained during operation; stricture of the
duodenal papilla was also found during operation and in 1 patient it had been
previously demonstrated by endoscopic cholangiography. The range of alkaline
phosphatase and transaminases is much the same as in common bile-duct obstruction from pancreas head tumour, although total bilirubin values are significantly lower.

The serial scintigram showed normal excretion patterns in 5 patients, a
delayed excretion in 8 patients and a complete obstruction in 3 patients. From
these latter patients, 2 showed a stricture in the duodenal papilla with an
impacted stone; the third patient was a 13-year old girl with multiple stones
in the biliary system and a biliary cirrhosis. Liver visualization in completely obstructed patients was good in 1 case (total bilirubin 325 µmol/l) and very
poor in the other 2 (total bilirubin respectively 306 and 600 µmol/l).
2 patients with a clinically active cholangitis showed a delayed excretion. No
significant differences were observed in the remaining patients, neither in the
clinical symptoms nor at operation, which explained the delayed or normal intestinal excretion. No visualization of the gall-bladder occurred in the patients
with stones in the gall-bladder. In 4 patients dilated bile-ducts were observed
on the serial images.

Time activity curves and functional images could be generated from 14
patients. In 2 patients with complete obstruction only blood-pool activity
could be seen. In table 9 the computer data are shown in comparison with bilirubin values and excretion patterns as observed on the serial scintigrams. It
can be seen from this table that only 2 patients show normal T max for the
right liver lobe; 3 patients show a normal T max for the left liver lobe and
only 1 patient shows normal T max for both lobes. In all other patients the uptake of the radiopharmaceutical by the liver is delayed; in 5 patients the
curve for the left liver lobe is ascending throughout the whole study. In spite
of the disturbed time activity curves for the uptake by the liver, the upslope
functional image was found to be normal for both liver lobes, except in 2
patients. One of these latter patients was also suffering from hyperlipaemia
and liver parenchyma involvement was possible; the other patient showed no
other indication of liver parenchyma disturbance.

With the exception of 2 patients in all patients the time activity curves
show a disturbed excretion for both right and left liver lobes; the curves show
a plateau for one or both liver lobes or show a continuous ascent for one of
the liver lobes. The downslope functional image was in agreement for the left

liver lobe; 1 patient with an abnormal curve for the right liver lobe showed
normal functional images. For 2 patients with a normal excretion curve for the
left liver lobe the downslope functional image was described as normal. From
this latter patient 1 patient showed an enlargement of the left liver lobe,
the other was known to have a slight liver function disturbance probably due to
medication with psychopharmaca.

Table 9. Maximum uptake time and half value time of the time activity curves of
16 patients with obstruction in common bile-duct in comparison with functional
imaging, bilirubin values and intestinal excretion observed on serial scintigram.

C= complete obstruction. D= delayed excretion. N= normal excretion. L= lengthened. P= plateau. AC= ascending curve. N= normal. A= abnormal. BPA= blood pool
activity.

total bilirubin µmol/l	intestinal excretion	T max right	T max left	T½ right	T½ left	upslope right	upslope left	downslope right	downslope left
46	D	18	23	P	P	N	N	A	A
23	D	26	AC	P	AC	N	A	N	A
119	D	32	AC	L	AC	N	A	A	A
70	D	30	16	L	P	N	N	A	A
306	C	BPA		BPA		BPA		BPA	
129	D	29	AC	P	AC	A	A	A	A
143	D	17	AC	L	AC	N	N	A	A
78	D	21	AC	L	AC	N	A	A	A
80	N	12	19	23	26	N	N	N	A
140	N	21	17	L	21	N	N	A	A
200	N	24	24	L	P	N	A	A	A
325	C	25	16	L	P	A	A	A	A
74	N	9	12	16	33	N	N	A	A
81	N	20	28	P	L	N	N	A	A
600	C	BPA		BPA		BPA		BPA	
100	D	28	36	L	P	A	A	A	A

In this group of patients 32 other investigations were performed. The
distribution of patients according to these parameters and success rate of
visualization of liver and/or bile-ducts is shown in table 10. In 3 of these
patients a liver biopsy was also carried out. 1 patient showed peritoneal
irritation after the biopsy. In 2 patients the biopsy indicated extrahepatic
obstruction. Oral cholecystography was performed when bilirubin values of 70
and 74 µmol/l were obtained; intravenous cholangiography was carried out in
cases with bilirubin values lower than 30 µmol/l. Abdominal plain film in 4
patients showed calcifications in the right upper abdomen, in all cases stones
were confirmed. The colloid liverscintigraphy was normal in 4 patients, 2

patients showed inhomogeneous distribution of the radioactivity and 1 patient
intrahepatic lesions due to (confirmed) liver cirrhosis.

Table 10. Clinical investigation in 16 patients with non-malignant obstruction
in bile-duct. Frequency of visualization of liver and/or bile-ducts.

| diagnostic investigation | no. patients | visualization of liver and/or bile-ducts | |
		success	failure
abdominal plain film	11	-	-
oral cholecystography	2	0	2
intravenous cholangiography	8	8	0
ultrasound study	4	4	0
colloid liver scintigraphy	7	7	0

The indication for a diagnosis of extrahepatic obstruction in intravenous
cholangiography is the visualization of dilated bile-ducts or stones in the
common bile-duct; with ultrasound study also dilated bile-duct should be shown.
In 8 patients IVC was performed; 6 showed patterns of extrahepatic obstruction.
In 5 cases common bile-duct stones were suspected. In 3 patients without stones
on the radiographic image - although a good visualization of the common bile-
duct was obtained - stones were found at operation. In only 1 case ultrasound
was suspect for extrahepatic obstruction. In none of these patients investigated
could stones in common bile-duct and gall-bladder be demonstrated by ultrasound.
In 2 cases the ultrasound study was suspect for a space occupying lesion in the
right liver lobe; these findings could not be confirmed. The results of the investigations are shown in table 11.

Table 11. Frequency of obstruction patterns in intravenous cholangiography,
ultrasound and cholescintigraphy; success rate in diagnosing extrahepatic obstruction.

diagnostic investigation	no. patients	dilated bile-ducts	stones in common bile-duct	intestinal excretion	correct diagnosis
intravenous cholangiography	8	6	5	-	5
ultrasound study	4	1	-		1
cholescintigraphy	16	4		14	16

Suspicion of extrahepatic obstruction on the cholescintigram, in the case of normal intestinal excretion, exists when bile-ducts appear dilated and time activity curves show a delayed excretion phase. In 1 patient none of these parameters were present and the findings by cholescintigraphy were indicative of delayed intestinal excretion due to parenchymal disease. However extra-hepatic obstruction by a process in the common bile-duct remained a possibility because there seemed to be an interruption in the common bile-duct on the serial scintigram . As can be seen from table 4, in all patients with delayed intestinal excretion, time activity curves from one or both liver lobes show a plateau after maximum uptake time has been reached or the curve continued to ascend during the whole study.

The results of the study of patients with obstructive jaundice due to a non-malignant obstruction of the common bile-duct showed the following patterns of cholescintigraphy.

Serial scintigraphy:

- normal intestinal excretion was observed in 31% of the patients studied
- delayed intestinal excretion was observed in 50%
- complete obstruction was observed in 19%.

In patients with a normal intestinal excretion dilated bile-ducts were observed in 80% and interruption in the common bile-duct in 20%. In 20% of the patients with a normal intestinal excretion a persistent slight blood-pool activity was observed. Patients with a complete obstruction showed:

- good liver visualization with persistence of slight blood-pool activity in 33% of the cases
- poor liver visualization with persistence of high blood-pool activity was observed in 67%.

In patients with a delayed intestinal excretion no persistent blood-pool activity was observed.

Computer data: No additional information could be obtained from the computer in 13% of the cases. Time activity curves obtained from patients with a normal intestinal excretion showed the following patterns:

- normal T max for both liver lobes in 20%
- delayed T max for both liver lobes in 20%
- normal T max for right liver lobe and delayed T max for left lobe 20%
- delayed T max for right lobe and normal T max for left lobe 40%
- normal $T\frac{1}{2}$ for both lobes in 40%
- lengthened $T\frac{1}{2}$ right lobe and normal $T\frac{1}{2}$ for left lobe 20%

- lengthened T½ for right lobe and plateau curve for left lobe 20%
- plateau curve for right lobe and lengthened T½ for left lobe 20%.

Time activity curves obtained from patients with delayed intestinal excretion showed the following patterns:

- delayed T max for right liver lobe in 100%
- delayed T max for left liver lobe in 38%
- lengthened T½ for right liver lobe in 62%
- the curve showed a plateau for right liver lobe in 38%
- the curve showed a plateau for left liver lobe in 38%
- continuously ascending curve for left liver lobe in 62%.

Time activity curves obtained from the patient with a complete obstruction showed the following patterns:

- delayed T max for the right liver lobe and normal for the left liver lobe
- lengthened T½ for right liver lobe while the curve showed a plateau for the left lobe.

Functional images obtained in all the patients studied revealed the following patterns:

- upslope images were normal for both liver lobes in 50% and normal for the right liver lobe alone in 29%; abnormal for both liver lobes in 21% and abnormal for the left liver lobe alone in 29%.
- downslope images were disturbed for both liver lobes in 86% and disturbed for the left liver lobe only in 14%.

Clinical reliability: Extrahepatic obstruction could be diagnosed if there was a complete obstruction on the serial scintigram, or if there was a visualization of dilated bile-ducts, or if there was a clear interruption in the common bile-duct. On the basis of these parameters extrahepatic obstruction was diagnosed on the serial scintigram alone in 50%. Extrahepatic obstruction could be found by the analysis of the computer data if time activity curves for one or both of the liver lobes showed a plateau or continued ascending during the whole study.

When serial scintigraphy patterns were combined with the results of the computer data the overall success rate for cholescintigraphy in diagnosing extrahepatic obstruction in this group of patients was 100%. Identification of dilated bile-ducts on the serial scintigram is a finding that be dependent on the experience of the investigator; the computer study is therefore necessary in these cases to diagnoze extrahepatic obstruction. In this group of patients the success rate forms intravenous cholangiography in diagnosing extrahepatic obstruction was 63% and for ultrasound 25%.

A typical case history is shown by the following example: A 76-years old female was admitted because of slight jaundice associated with pain in right upper abdomen radiating to the back and coupled with nausea and vomiting. A cholecystectomy had been performed some time before. On physical examination the patient had slight jaundice and an enlarged liver lobe palpable in the middle abdomen.

Laboratory findings:	total bilirubin 50 μmol/l, direct reacting bilirubin 15.2 μmol/l, alkaline phosphatase 500 mU/ml, SGOT 13 mU/ml, SGPT 26 mU/ml
intravenous cholangiography:	visualized a dilated common bile-duct with large aberrations in diameter. There were no distinct indications for concrements.
cholescintigraphy	
serial scintigraphy: (fig. 2-14)	an enlarged liver, especially the left lobe which also showed reduced uptake of activity. Distended intrahepatic bile-ducts with interruption in common bile-duct; normal excretion into the intestine. The gall-bladder was not visualized.
time activity curves: (fig. 2-15)	normal uptake and excretion in right liver lobe, a normal uptake in left liver lobe, but a delayed excretion
cumulative image: (fig. 2-16)	dilated intrahepatic bile-ducts and interruption of common bile-duct
functional images: (fig. 2-16)	upslope image shows disturbed uptake in left liver lobe and in the caudal part of the right liver lobe. Downslope image shows disturbed excretion in left liver lobe and in the caudal part of the right liver lobe.
conclusion:	suspected of obstruction in common bile-duct; liver parenchyma is slightly disturbed
surgery:	a congested liver was found (caused by decompensated heart) with slight dilated bile-ducts and a stone in the common bile duct.

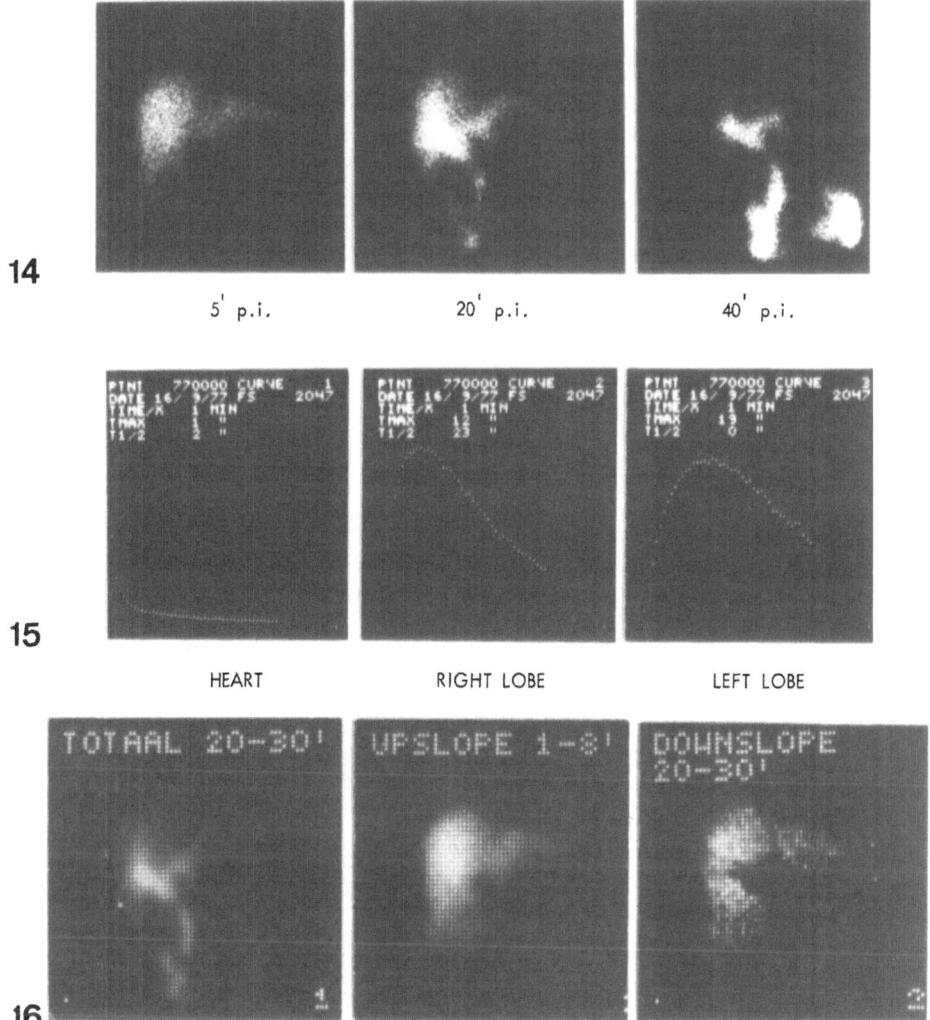

14

5' p.i.   20' p.i.   40' p.i.

15

HEART   RIGHT LOBE   LEFT LOBE

16

A 84-year old female was admitted with jaundice and pain in right upper abdomen.

Laboratory findings:	total bilirubin 140 μmol/l, direct reacting bilirubin 99 μmol/l, alkaline phosphatase 440 mU/ml, SGOT 33 mU/ml, SGPT 47 mU/ml
abdominal plain film:	calcification in the right upper abdomen
intravenous cholangiography: (performed when total bili- rubin level fall to 26 umol/l)	a grossly dilated common bile-duct with poor definition and no gall-bladder
cholescintigraphy	
serial scintigraphy: (fig. 3-20)	good visualization of the liver with dilata- tion of intrahepatic bile ducts and common bile-duct; no visualization of gall-bladder but normal intestinal excretion
time activity curves: (fig. 3-21)	delayed uptake by the right liver lobe with a delayed excretion. The uptake in the left liver lobe was normal but the excretion was delayed.
functional images: (fig. 3-22)	normal uptake by right and left lobe with a good image of the common bile-duct on the image from 26 - 35'. The downslope functional image is diffusely inhomogeneous, confirming that the excretion phase of the whole liver is disturbed.
conclusion:	suspected bile-duct obstruction; liver paren- chyma disturbance
surgery:	multiple stones in gall-bladder and common bile-duct were demonstrated. Passage to the duodenum was poor.
peroperative cholangiography:	grossly dilated common bile-duct with multiple stones

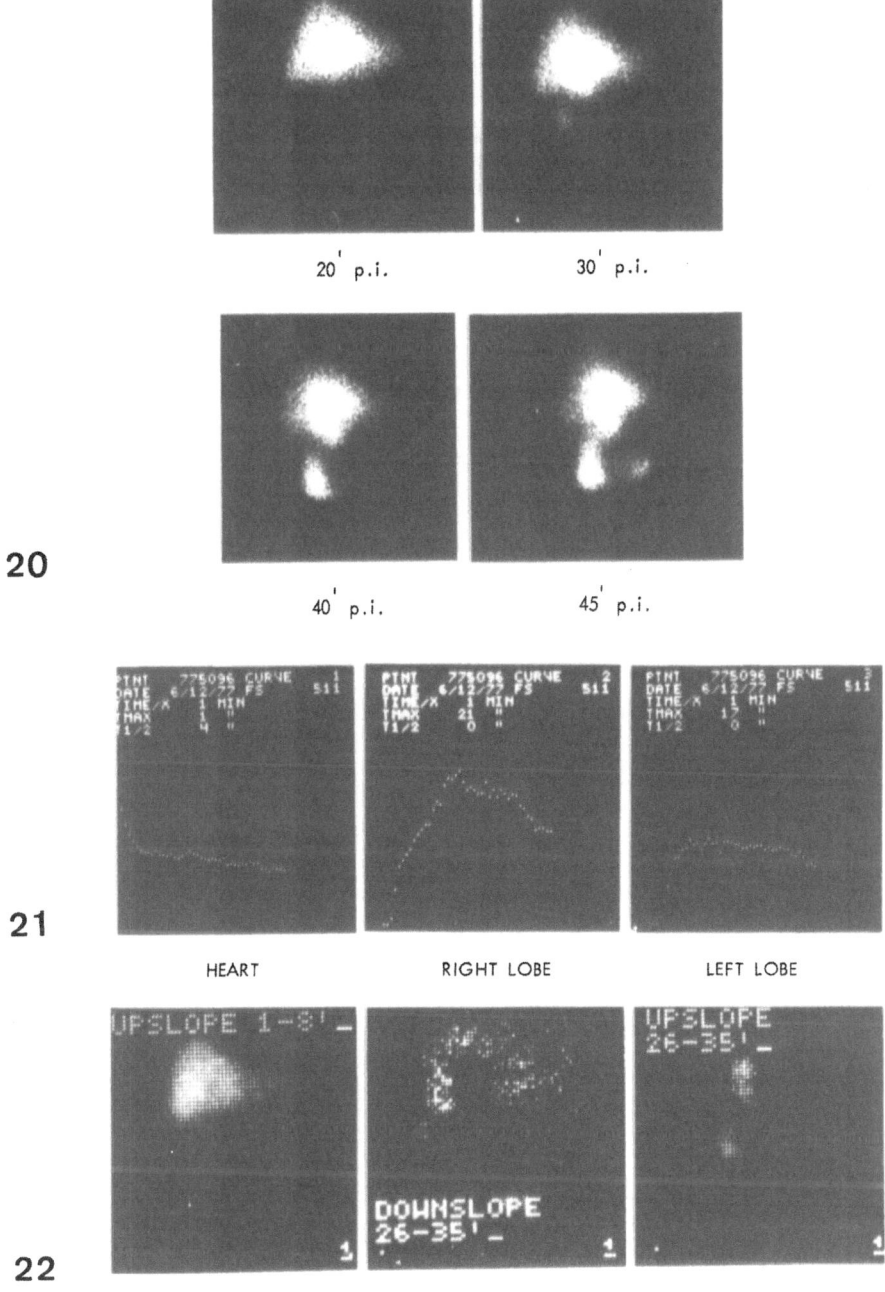

20' p.i.   30' p.i.

20

40' p.i.   45' p.i.

21

HEART   RIGHT LOBE   LEFT LOBE

22

REFERENCES

1. Pors Nielsen S et al, Hepatobiliary scintigraphy and hepatography with Tc^{99m}-Diethylacetanilido iminodiacetate in obstructive jaundice. J. nucl. Med. 19:452, 1978.

2. Fueger GF, Differential diagnosis of hepatocellular and obstructive jaundice. In: Hepatobiliary scintigraphy by means of Ida-derivatives. Biersack HJ, Mahlstedt J (eds), Stuttgart, G-I-T/E Giebeler, 1978.

3. Wolf F, Complete and incomplete obstruction. Ibid.

4. Pedersen SA et al, Hepatobiliary scintigraphy with ^{99m}Tc Ida and ^{99m}Tc Sulphur colloid. Comparison of abilities to demonstrate biliary obstruction and hepatic metastases. Eur. J. Nucl. Med. 3:305, 1980

5. Tjen HSLM, Cox PH, The use of ^{99m}Tc diethylida combined with functional imaging for the differentiation of obstructive and functional jaundice. In: Nuklear Medizin - Clinical value of nuclear methods. Schmidt HAE, Ortiz Berrocal J, Stuttgart, Schattauer, 1979.

6. Dudzak R et al, Clinical application of ^{99m}Tc labelled ida derivatives. In: Nuklear Medizin. Nuclear Medicine with its interdependencies. Schmidt HAE, Wolf F (eds), Stuttgart, Schattauer (in print) 1980.

7. Tjen HSLM, Cholescintigraphy. Ph.D. Thesis, University of Utrecht, The Netherlands (in English), 1979.

9. CHOLESCINTIGRAPHY IN FOCAL LIVER DISEASE

H.J. BIERSACK

9.1. INTRODUCTION

The detection and evaluation of space-occupying lesions in the liver is usually not performed using hepatobiliary scintigraphy with Ida-derivatives. The method of choice here is colloid-scintigraphy. In a few cases Ida-scintigraphy can yield additional information for differential diagnosis respectively to check on the proliferation of malignancy. The results obtained by these methods are discussed below for different focal liver processes.

9.2. Hepatic Adenoma

It is known that hepatic adenomas can accumulate radiocolloids. Ameriks et al (1), Motsay et al (2), Sackett et al (3) and Lerona et al (4) described negative colloid-scintigraphies in the presence of important focal lesions, whereas Salvo et al (5) illustrate a large number of cases where hepatic adenoma causes accumulation defects. Casarella et al (6) correlated arteriographic findings with colloid-scintigraphy and found accumulation defects of colloids in the case of hypo-vascularization, which is frequently found in hepatic adenoma.

Functional liver scintigraphy findings with hepatic adenomas are encountered only twice in the literature: Sackett et al (3) describe the accumulation of both radiocolloid and 131-I Rose Bengal. Belfer et al (7) report a case of hepatic adenoma, developing as the result of oral contraceptive usage. In this case the adenoma showed an accumulation of Tc^{99m} Diethylida whereas Tc^{99m} sulfur colloid showed an accumulation defect. In the majority of cases hepatic adenomas appears to be characterized by colloid accumulation defects in the scintigram, in contrast to focal nodular hyperplasia. The findings made so far with hepatobiliary scintigraphy are still too scattered to allow a general conclusion about the behaviour of radiopharmaceuticals for cholescintigraphy in the presence of this type of liver-tumour to be made.

9.3. Nodular focal lesions

According to the literature nodular focal lesions (NFL) are characterized
in most cases by accumulation defects (5), although normal scintigrams were
found also in cases where the presence of large focal lesions was confirmed
postoperatively (8,9) which is evidence in favour of accumulation in the lesion.
Cases of increased local accumulation in NFL have also been described (5,10,11).
Casarella et al (6) again found a correlation between the accumulation of sulphur
colloid in the NFL with a hypervascularization.

Only three cases have been described so far with Ida-derivatives (12). In
a case with a normal colloid scintigram a neatly defined activity retention in
the NFL was found probably because of proliferation of the bile ducts (13)
(fig. 1). Another patient had a focal accumulation failure in the colloid-
scintigram as well as on the Ida-scintigram (fig. 2). In a third case both Ida
and colloids accumulated in the NFL (fig. 3). I-131 labeled Rose Bengal was also
used in patients with NFL (14,15). In both reports functional scintigraphy
showed accumulation defects. These results demonstrate that sulfur colloid liver
scanning in combination with functional Ida-scintigraphy can be helpful in the
diagnosis of NFL when the lesion has functioning liver parenchyma which can be
indentified. However, the variability of the findings indicated that NFL can be
regarded as the "sphinx" of liver tumours, since they contribute little or
nothing to the resolution of the confusion which results from the "myriad of
diagnostic terms pathologists have used to refer to focal nodular hyperplasia"
(6) (figs. 1,2,3).

9.4. Hepatoma

The first publication concerning a combined colloid and functional scintigram in the presence of hepatocellular carcinoma was made by Hebestreit et al
(16). The colloid-scintigram showed an accumulation defect, whereas the Ida-
scintigraphy demonstrated accumulation of the tracer in a histologically
confirmed liver cell carcinoma. Ueno and Haseda (17) also observed accumulation
of a cholescintigraphic radiopharmaceutical: an accumulation defect on the
colloid-scintigram in parallel to an accumulation and excretion of Tc^{99m}-Pyri-
doxilidene Isoleucin in a hepatoma. In contrast, Kroiss et al (18) found, in
all of his patients with hepatocellular carcinoma, focal accumulation defects
in the Ida-scintigram and emphasized the value of the information obtained about
the extrahepatic bile ducts. Cannon et al (19) also reported an accumulation
defect on a Tc^{99m}-Pipida-scintigram in a case of hepatoma with pulmonary

metastases. In this exceptional case the Ida-derivative accumulated in radio-
logically confirmed pulmonary metastases.

9.5. Liver metastases

There have been sporadic reagents of the value of Ida-scintigraphy in liver
metastases. Pedersen et al (20) point out that Ida and colloid-scintigraphy
complement each other well in biliary obstruction where there is suspicion of
liver metastases, because accumulation defects in the colloid-scintigram are
frequently observed as result of bile stasis. In these cases hepatobiliary
scintigraphy allows the classification of accumulation defects due to stasis,
thus eliminating the possible presence of metastases. In addition, functional
liver-scintigraphy allows the visualization of bile-duct and gall-bladder
displacement prior to compensatory surgery in the event of liver metastases
(fig. 4).

9.6. Benign liver tumours

Occasionally hepatobiliary scintigraphy may be of value for the differential diagnosis of liver (echinococcus) cysts. An example is shown in fig. 5 where
in a patient with liver echinococcus, suspected of having a gall-bladder-hydrops
on the basis of an ultrasound diagnosis, bile-duct-scintigraphy demonstrated an
intrahepatic space-occupying lesion with desplacement of the gall-bladder.
Functional scintigraphy hence corrected and complemented the ultrasound investigation.

9.7. Liver trauma

The first report concerning the use of cholescintigraphy with Tc^{99m}-ida
in liver trauma appeared in 1979 (21) in a case history concerning a bile-duct
rupture. In 1967, Spencer et al (22) and later Wiener and Vyas (23) and Zaw-win
et al (24), had already reported on the use of I-131 Rose Bengal for the
detection of biliary fistula. The method is simple and non-invasive, and permits
the determination of the extent, localization and spread of bile leakage. This
is particularly important because the early detection of a bile-duct rupture
can reduce the incidence of mortality. Sty et al (25) reported a case of liver
trauma in which Ida-scintigraphy facilitated the detection of bile-leakage into
liver tissue and the peritoneal cavity. Since every liver trauma can be
accompanied by a bile-duct rupture, non-invasive cholscintigraphy should be used
as a screening method. Postoperative cholescintigraphy can be used also to

obtain information about accidential ligature of the bile-ducts (fig.6),
facilitating puncture of the bile-ducts under stasis during PTC .

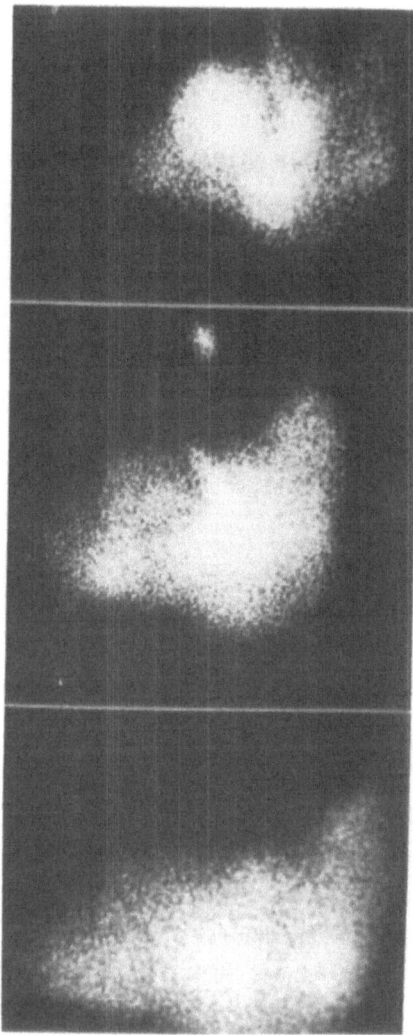

Fig. 1. FNH of the liver:
a) Liverscan with Tc^{99m}-Sulfur colloid: inhomogenous uptake but no circumscribed defect.
b,c) Liver-scintigraphy with Tc^{99m}-Ida: impaired excretion of the tracer in
circumscribed areas of both liver lobes.

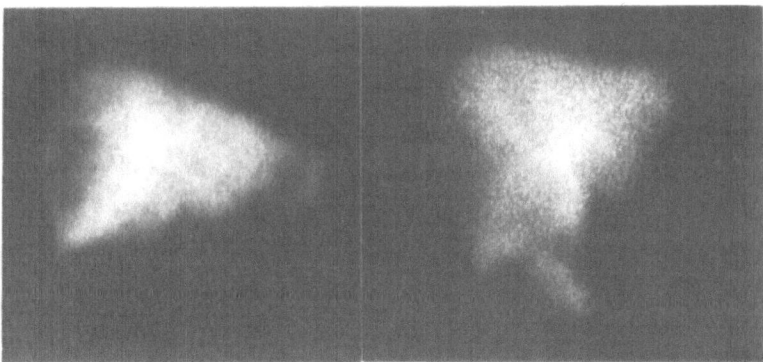

Fig. 2. FNH of the liver:
a) Liverscan with Tc^{99m}-Sulfur colloid: large multilobular filling defect in the right liver lobe.
b) Liver-scintigraphy with Tc^{99m}-Ida: no accumulation of the tracer by FNH.

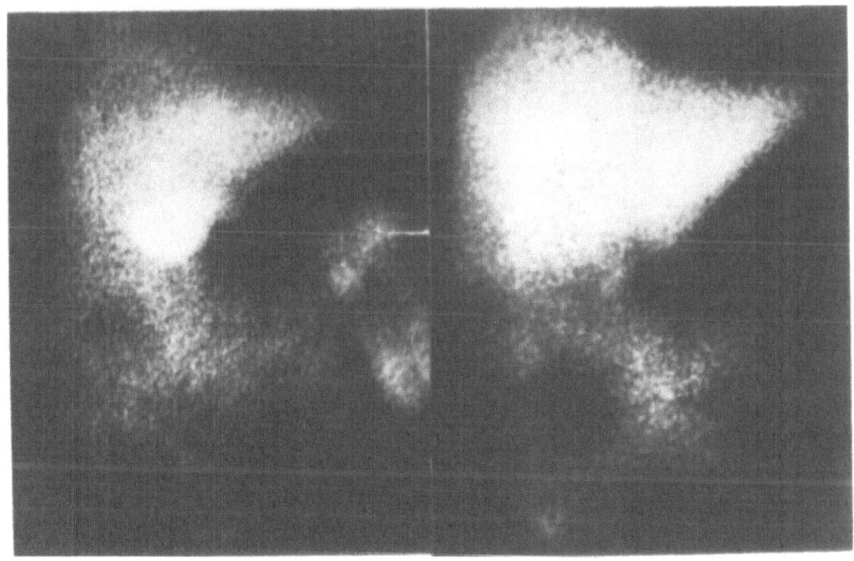

Fig. 3. FNH of the liver:
a) Liverscan with Tc^{99m}-Sulfur colloid.
b) Liver-scintigraphy with Tc^{99m}-Ida: uptake of both tracers within FNH.

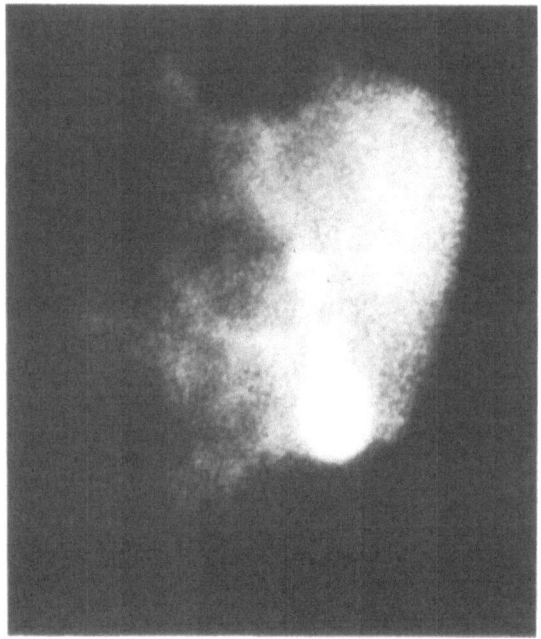

Fig. 4. Liver-scintigraphy with Tc^{99m}-Ida in liver metastases: clearcut visualization of the gall-bladder before puncture.

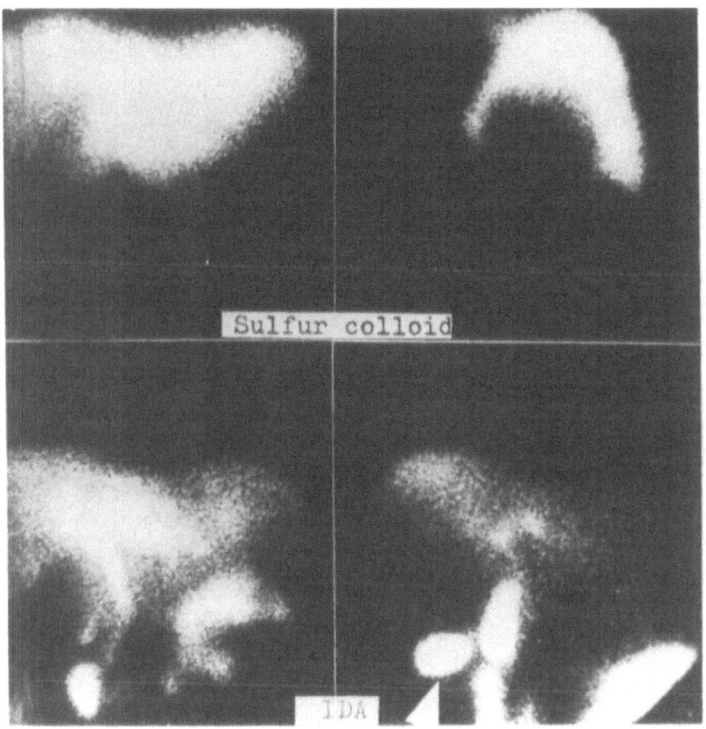

Fig. 5. Hydatide cyste of the liver:
a) Liverscan with Tc^{99m}-Sulfur colloid (left: anterior, right: lateral)
b) Liver-scintigraphy with Tc^{99m}-Ida: displacement of the gall-bladder by the cyst.

146

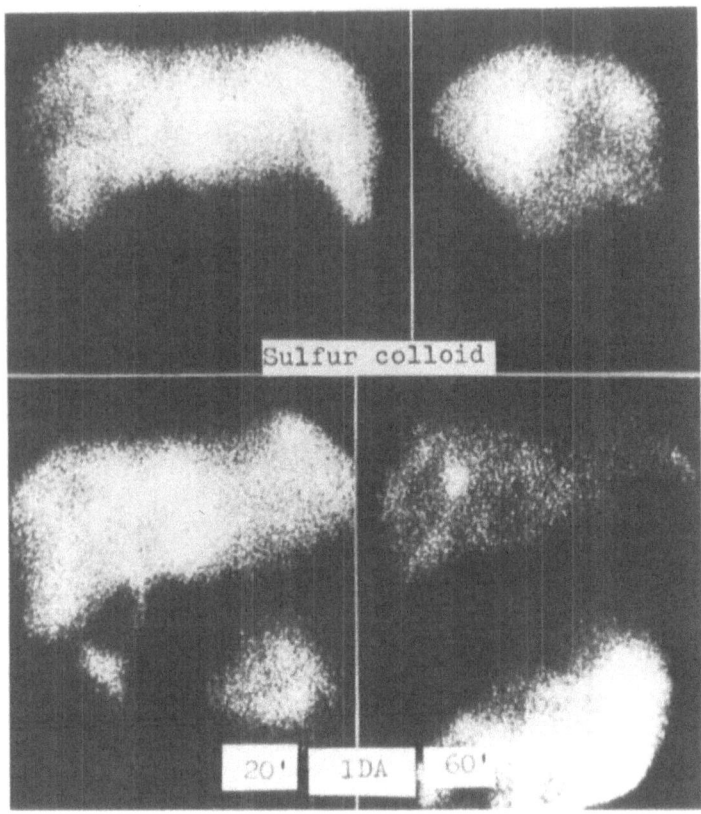

Fig. 6. Accidental ligature of the right hepatic duct after surgery because of liver rupture:
a) Liverscan with Tc^{99m}-Sulfur colloid.
b) Liver-scintigraphy with Tc^{99m}-Ida: dilated bile-ducts in the right liver lobe, regular bile discharge from the left lobe.

REFERENCES

1. Ameriks JA, Thompson NW, Frey CW, Hepatic cell adenomas, spontaneous liver rupture and oral contraceptives. Arch. Surg. 110:548, 1975.

2. Motsay G, Gamble WG, Clinical experience with hepatic adenomas. Surg. Gynec. Obstet. 134:415, 1972.

3. Sackett J, Mosenthol W, House R, Scintillation scanning of liver cell adenoma. Amer. J. Roentgenol. 113:56, 1971.

4. Lerona PT, Go RT, Cornell SH, Limitations of angiography and scanning in diagnosis of liver masses. Radiology 112:139, 1974.

5. Salvo AF, Schiller A, Athanasoulis C, Hepatoadenoma and focal nodular hyperplasia: Pitfalls in radiocolloid imaging. Radiology 125:451, 1977.

6. Casarella WJ, Knowles DM, Wolff M, Focal nodular hyperplasia and liver cell adenoma: Radiologic and pathologic differentiation. Amer. J. Roentgenol. 131:393, 1978.

7. Belfer AJ, Grijm R, Van der Schoot JB, Hepatic adenoma: Imaging with different radionuclides. Clin. Nucl. Med. 4:375, 1979.

8. McLoughlin MJ, Gilday DL, Angiography and colloid scanning of benign mass lesions of the liver. Clin. Radiol. 23:377, 1972.

9. Zurbriggen S, Tylén U, Angiographische Befunde bei fokaler nodulärer Hyperplasie der Leber. Röfo 122:404, 1975.

10. Pasquier J, Dorta T, Focal hyperfixation of radiocolloid by the liver (letter). J. nucl. Med. 15:725, 1974.

11. Jhingram S, Mukhopadhyay A, Ajmani S, Hepatic adenomas and focal nodular hyperplasia of the liver in young women on oral contraceptives: Case reports. J. nucl. Med. 18:263, 1977.

12. Biersack HJ, Thelen M, Torres JF, Focal nodular hyperplasia of the liver as established by $99m$Tc Sulfurcolloid and HIDA scintigraphy. Radiology 137:187, 1980.

13. Knowles DM, Wolff M, Focal nodular hyperplasia of the liver. A clinicopathologigic study and review of the literature. Human Pathology 7:533, 1976.

14. Wilson TS, MacGregor JW, Focal nodular hyperplasia of the liver: the solitary cirrhotic liver nodule. Canad. Med. Ass. J. 100:567, 1969.

15. McMullen CT, Montgomery JL, Angiographic findings of focal nodular hyperplasia of the liver and review of the literature. Amer. J. Roentgenol. 117:380, 1973.

16. Hebestreit HP, Böttger E, Trede M, Szintigraphische Diagnose einer primären Leberzellkarzinoms mit einem neuen Radiopharmazeutikum. Röfo 127:486, 1977.

17. Ueno K, Haseda Y, Concentration and clearance of $99m$Tc-pyridoxylidene isoleucine by a hepatoma. Clin. Nucl. Med. 5:196, 1980.

18. Kroiss A, Weiss W, Peschl L, $99m$Tc-Hepatobida-Untersuchungen bei Leberparenchymdefekten. In: Nuklearmedizin - Klinische Bedeutung nuklearmedizinischer Diagnostik und Therapie, Riccabona G, Schmidt HAE (eds), Stuttgart, New York, Schattauer.

19. Cannon JR, Long RF, Berens SV, Uptake of $99m$Tc-Pipida in pulmonary metastases from a hepatoma. Clin. Nucl. Med. 5:22, 1978.

148

20. Pedersen SA, Øster-Jørgensen E, Schoubye J, Hepatobiliary scintigraphy with [99mTc]-Hida and [99mTc]-Sulfur colloid. Comparison of the abilities to demonstrate biliary obstruction and hepatic metastases. Eur. J. Nucl. Med. 5:305, 1980.

21. Weissmann HS, Chun KJ, Frank M, Demonstration of traumatic bile leakage with cholescintigraphy and ultrasonography. Amer. J. Roentgenol. 133:843, 1979.

22. Spencer RP, Marshall MK, Glenn WL, Use of [131]I- Rose Bengal to follow bile leakage. Amer. J. dig. Dis. 12:1169, 1967.

23. Wiener SN, Vyas M, The scintigraphic demonstration of bile leakage utilizing ^{131}I-Rose Bengal. J. nucl. Med. 15:1044, 1974.

24. Zaw-win B, Darwish M, Dibos PE, ^{131}I-Rose Bengal scanning in the detection of cholecystocolic fistula. Amer. J. Gastroent. 68:396, 1977.

25. Sty JR, Babbitt DP, Squires W, Tc-99mIda hepatobiliary imaging: a fractured liver. Clin. Nucl. Med. 4:493, 1979.

10. EXAMINATION OF PATIENTS WITH BILIODIGESTIVE ANASTOMOSES

H.G. REICHELT

10.1.DEFINITION

Biliodigestive anastomoses are operatively reconstructed connecting passages between parts of the bile-draining system and parts of the upper digestive tract - essentially the duodenum and the jejunum - to guarantee an unhindered bile flow.

10.2.Surgical techniques

At the present time surgical techniques are in use:
- side-to-side choledochoduodenostomy
- hepaticoduodenostomy
- cholecystoduodenostomy
- cholesystojejunostomy
- end-to-side (resp. end-to-end) choledocho- hepaticojejunostomy with retro-antecolic Roux-en-Y-loop
- hepatico- jejuno- duodenostomy (Grassi)
- high biliodigestive anastomoses (with or without transanastomotic drains)
- hepaticojejunostomy in the hilus
- intrahepatic hepaticojejunostomy (Coinaud-Hepp)

Of all the possible procedures at present in use to procedure biliodigestive anastomoses preference will be given in this report to choledocho- hepatico-jejunostomy in benigne diseases and to choledocho- cholecystoduodenostomy in malignant diseases.

10.3.Postoperative complications and sequelae associated with biliodigestive anastomoses

Postoperative complications. Early postoperative complications particularly occur following the difficult placement of biliodigestive anastomoses high in the liver hilus and when a tender common bile duct and/or hepatic duct is present. Mainly there are to be expected:

- suture insufficiency (fig. 3)
- primary blockage (figs. 4,5) or:
- considerable stenosis of the anastomosis due to primary narrowing caused by
  the suture of postsurgical edema (fig. 6).

     Occasionally the diagnosis of these disorders is difficult in so far as a
postoperative choleperitonitis may take an imperceptible turn and jaundice may
be referred to the previous biliary duct obstruction.

<u>Sequelae after biliodigestive anastomoses</u>

     Secondary stenosis of the anastomoses (figs 7,8) and cholangitis are
the main complications which may often manifest themselves years after surgery.
Between both there is an interaction. Stenosis leads to bile congestion and
cholangitis. Cholangitis initiates further shrinking of the anastomosis
especially in the case of high anastomoses. The significance of the reflux of
chyme into the bile ducts by a wide anastomosis is still controversial. The
question is, whether or not a reflux of chyme will cause a cholangitis when the
anastomosis is of sufficient width and the connected part of the digestive tract
shows an adequate motility. Long term observations show that a reflux is always
a potential hazard and mostly leads to a manifest damage due to cholangitis. The
situation is changed for the worse when the segment of the intestine distal to
the anastomosis functions as "blind loop". The choledocho- hepaticojejunostomy
has an advantage over other kinds of anastomoses in that the long (40-60 cm),
isoperistaltically disengaged loop safely prevents the reflux of ingesta into
the biliary tract. This method is even superior to the "omega"-loop, which does
not exclude reflux.

10.4.<u>Causes of postoperative complications with secondary liver cell damage:</u>
- stenosis of the anastomosis in preoperative normal bile ducts (1-15.5%)
- preceding strictures along bile ducts (30-40%)
- impaired drainage due to the Roux-en-Y-loop "blind loop" syndrome or
  "strangulation phenomenon" (fig. 9). Such syndromes are well-known in the
  literature, but morbidity ratios are not reliably documented.

10.5.Problems associated with current diagnostic procedures

     The investigation of complaints and symptoms after biliodigestive anastomo-
ses have been created requires an exact biomedical and enzyme evaluation of liver
function and especially examinations of the width of the anastomosis as well as

of the transport conditions in the anastomized loop. So far radiology has
played the major role in evaluating the function of biliodigestive anastomoses:

Abdominal plain film may show air in the biliary tract. Air in the bile
ducts is ample evidence, that the anastomosis is open, but does not give
adequate confirmation of the sufficiency of the anastomosis. Additional information is always necessary.

The barium meal occasionally helps in the assessment of anastomosis function
and reflux in choledocho- hepaticoduodenostomy and in choledochohepaticojejuno-
stomy with an "omega"-loop (fig. 2). Prognostic statements about biliodigestive
anastomoses using the Roux-en-Y-loop technique are not possible.

Intravenous infusion cholangiography may occasionally detect an initial
stenosis in a biliodigestive anastomosis, however, in the presence of impaired
liver function (e.g. chronic cholangitis) the procedure gives insufficient
information. Intravenous infusion cholangiography is ineffective when the bilirubin levels increase above 4 mg/100 ml. A diagnostic evaluation of the function
of Roux-en-Y-loop is not feasible.

Endoscopic retrograde cholangiography (ERC) is only of diagnostic value with
choledocho- hepaticoduodenostomy.

Percutaneous transhepatic cholangiography (PTC) should be applied with
caution with respect to the cholangitis which is usually present. In addition
particularly in the presence of chronic cholangitis the procedure is technically
difficult to perform.

Ultrasound can not rule out obstruction in the presence of chronic
cholangitis and it is not possible to evaluate the functional behaviour of the
draining loop.

10.6. Cholescintigraphy
    Method. The fasting (no strict requirement) patient is investigated in
supine position with the gamma camera head placed over the liver and the
abdomen.

Radiopharmaceutical: Diethyl-Ida 5-10 mCi intravenously.

Imaging protocol. Serial scintigrams are recorded at 5 minutes intervals until 30 minutes post injection. Additional scintigrams are made 45, 60 and 90 minutes post injection. When no intestinal activity is seen at this time and no intrahepatic ducts show up scintigrams are made at 2 hours intervals until 6 hours after injection to demonstrate delayed intestinal excretion or complete obstruction. It appears advisable to make scintiphotos in the upright or oblique position to induce activity flow in the anastomized loop and in order to get optimal information concerning the anatomic situation.

Time activity curves and retention indices. The digital information stored in a computer can be analyzed and time activity curves generated by selecting regions of interest for heart, right and left liver lobe. T max (time required until maximum activity is reached), T max/2 (time up to half maximum). The T max/2 cannot be measured during the normal period of study in every case due to prolonged retention time in liver disease and obstruction. The "uptake index" defined as the ratio of right liver lobe counts to cardiac counts at 3 minutes and 30 minutes after injection can be calculated. Time activity curves and retention indices are only valuable in follow-up studies to register changes in liver function.

10.7. Summary

Cholescintigraphy in evaluation of function of biliodigestive anastomoses has the following indisputable advantages:
- The procedure is noninvasive. The radiation burden can be neglected.
- Cholescintigraphy is effective even in patients with high bilirubin levels (up to 12 mg/100 ml).
- Stasis in intrahepatic bile ducts, incomplete and complete obstruction of the biliodigestive anastomosis are usually well recognized.
- Cholescintigraphy allows the investigation of the Roux-en-Y-loop and gives information on the functional behaviour.
- Cholescintigraphy is especially suitable for follow-up studies. The clinical usefulness of the technique can be improved by quantitative assessment of liver uptake and calculating retention indices.

Following points proved to be disadvantageous:
- The deliniation of anatomical details is insufficient.

- The diagnosis of obstruction in advanced destructing cholangitis is difficult
  or impossible.

These advantages can be minimized or overcome by taking into account the
detailed knowledge of the surgical procedure when setting up follow-up studies.

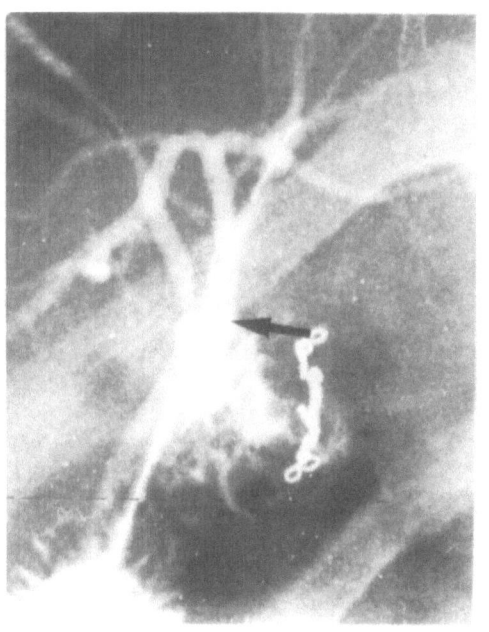

Fig. 1a

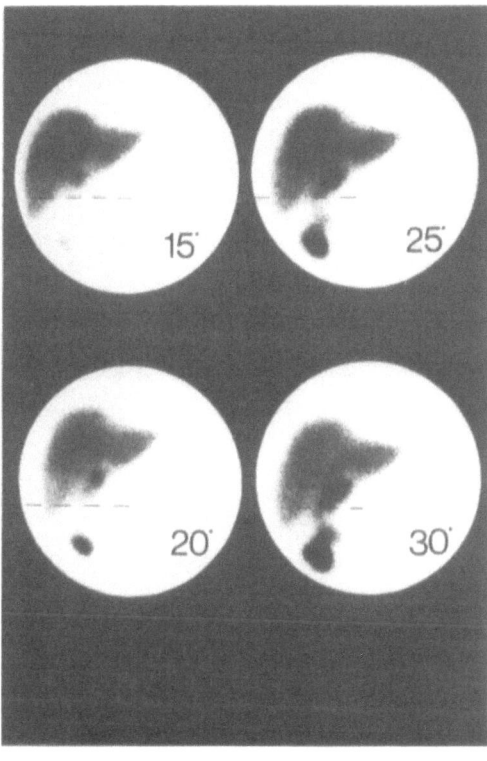

Fig. 1b

Fig. 1.   High hepaticojejunostomy; 1 year postoperative; bilirubin normal.
Fig. 1a shows the postoperative cholangiogram with a trans anastomotic drain;
normal width of anastomosis (◄—).

Fig. 1b. Cholescintigram: normal findings (— — — hiatus of mesocolon).

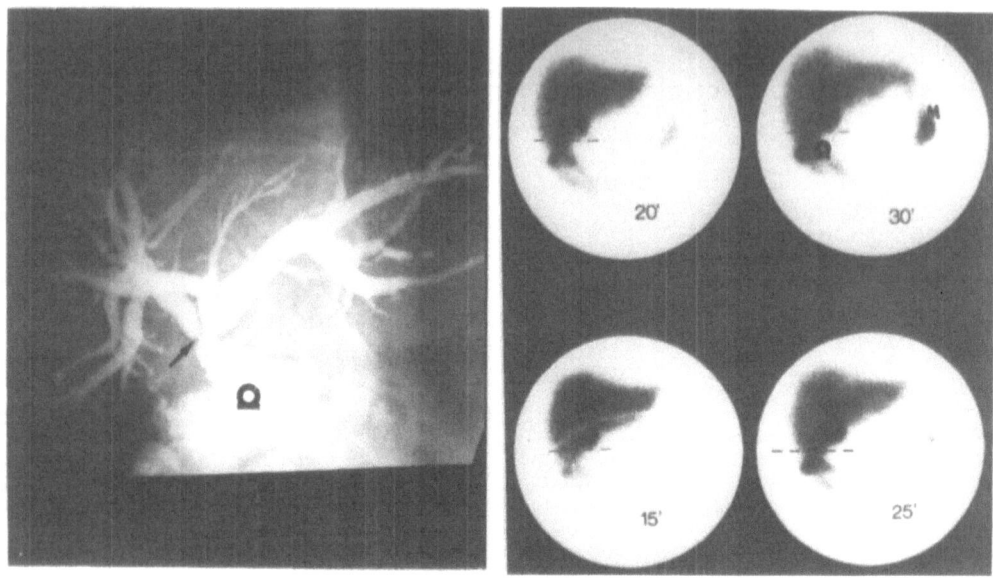

Fig. 2a   Fig. 2b

Fig. 2.   Hepaticojejunostomy with omega loop (Ω); 8 months postoperative;
right upper abdominal pain; bilirubin normal; cholangitis.

Fig. 2a. The barium meal shows an enormous barium reflex into the intrahepatic
bile ducts (◄— anastomosis).

Fig. 2b. Cholescintigram: no obstruction; good visualisation of the omega loop
(M stomach).

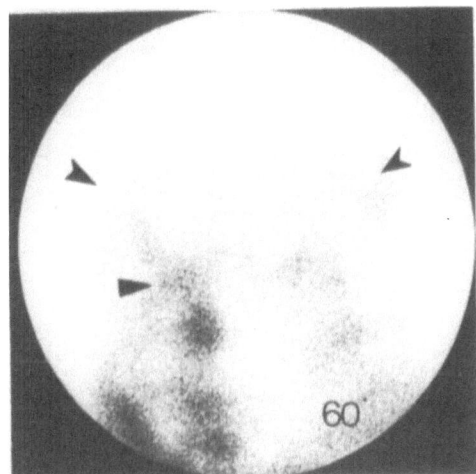

Fig. 3. Intraperitoneal bile fistula following choledochojejunostomy; Cholescintigram: increased background activity only in the peritoneal cavity,
deliniated by diaphragm, (◄); activity in bile ducts (◄) and bowel.

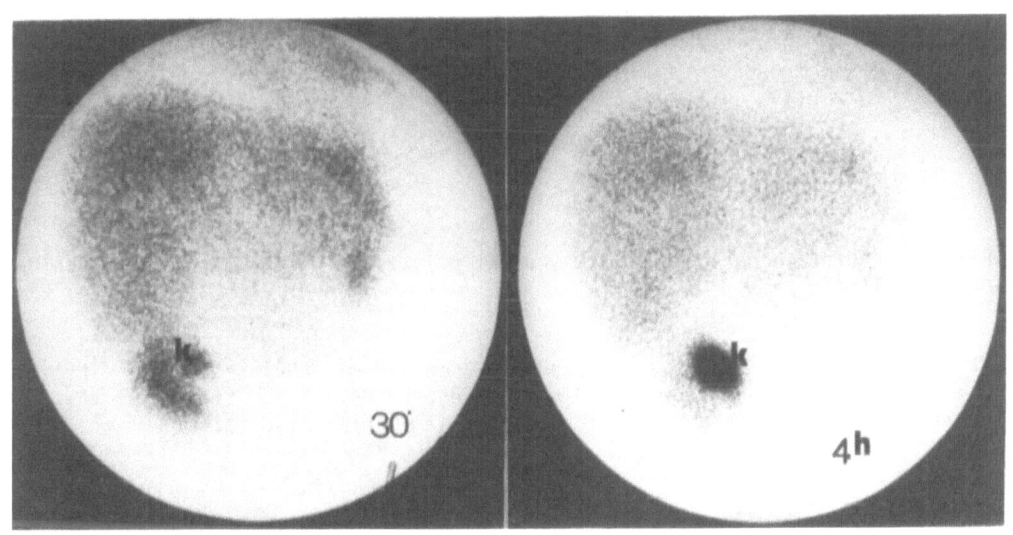

Fig. 4a   Fig. 4b

Fig. 4a. Livertransplant - complete obstruction of anastomosis; bilirubin 12 mg/
100 ml.

Fig. 4a,b. Cholescintigram (30 min and 4 hr): no activity in praeanastomotic bile
ducts and in the bowel up to 4 hr; heterotopic elimination of the radiopharmaceutical by the kidney (K right kidney).

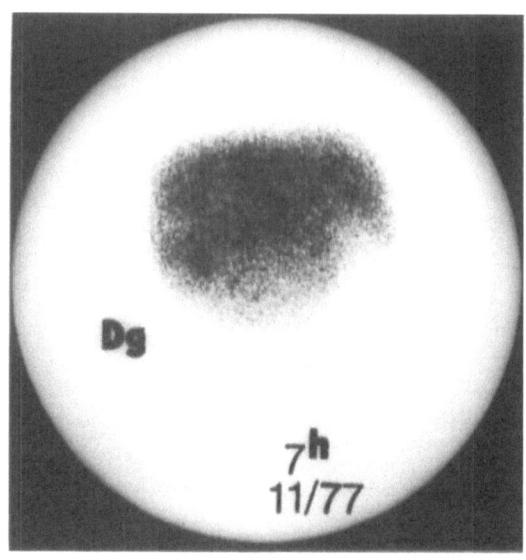

Fig. 5a

Fig. 5a. (Left)- hepaticojejunostomy after polytrauma with complete destruction
of right liver lobe.

Fig. 5a. Increasing jaundice; bilirubin 6,5 mg/100 ml. Cholescintigram (7hr):
complete obstruction of the biliodigestive anastomosis - no activity in the
bowel up to 7 hr; transanastomotic drainage (Dg minimally effective).

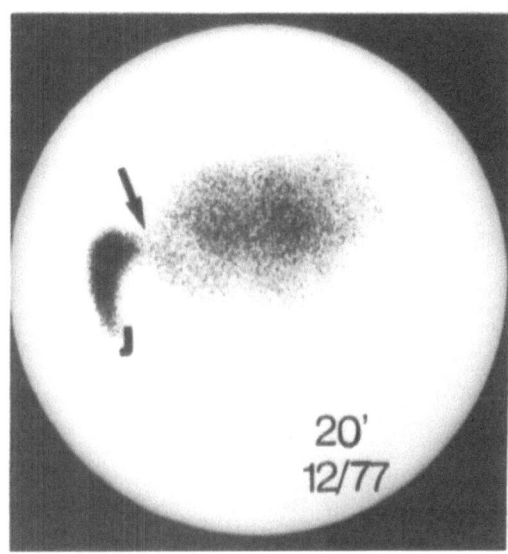

Fig. 5b

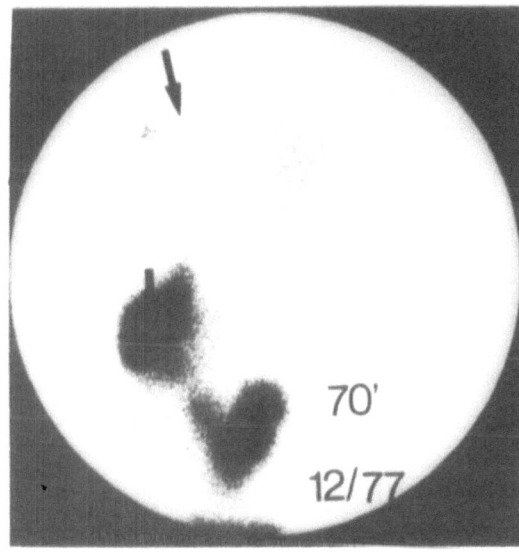

Fig. 5c

Fig. 5b,c. Reconstruction of the hepaticojejunostomy; bilirubin 2 mg/100 ml
2 weeks postoperative. Cholescintigram (20 min and 70 min): free bile flow into
the jejunum (J) (← anastomosis).

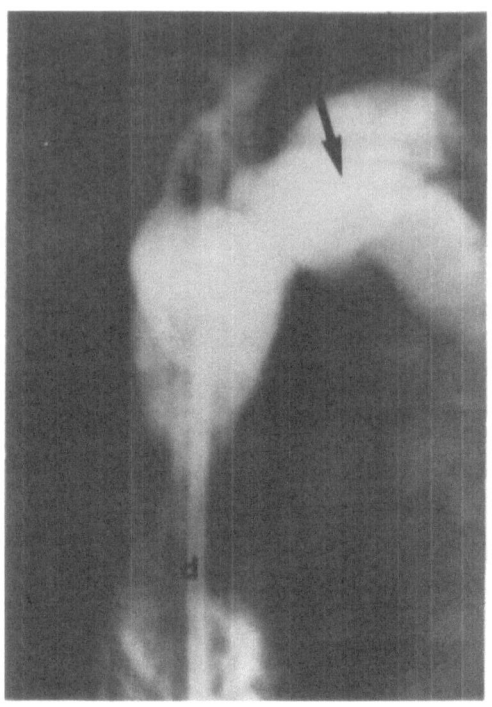

Fig. 6a

Fig. 6a. Choledochojejunostomy - primary narrowing suture; bilirubin 1,5 mg/ 100 ml.

Fig. 6a. Cholangiogram via transanastomotic drain (d) shows narrow anastomosis (◄); preoperative dilated left intrahepatic duct (←).

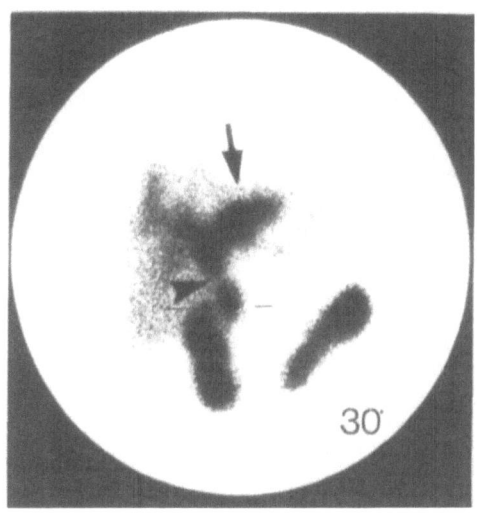

Fig. 6b

Fig. 6b. Cholescintigram (30 min): intensively filled intrahepatic ducts -
stenosis at the anastomosis.

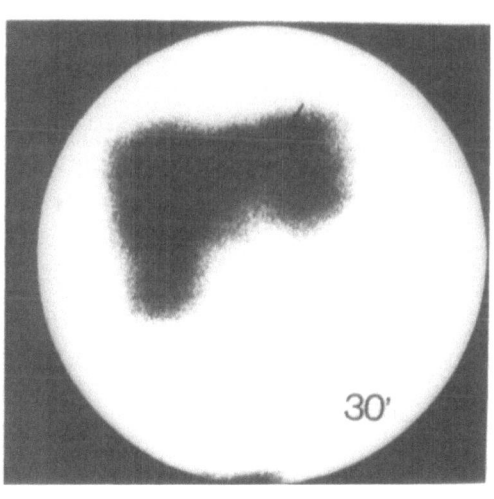

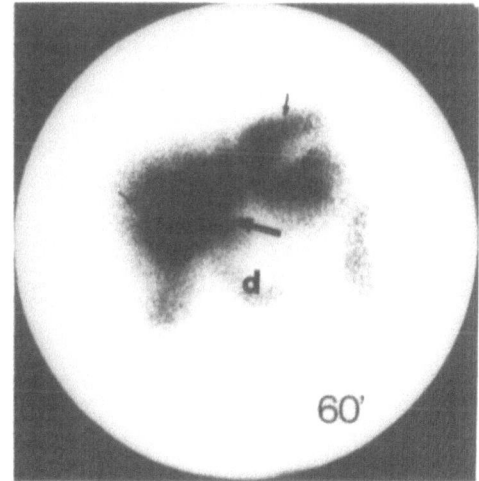

Fig. 7a

Fig. 7b

Fig. 7a. Choledochoduodenostomy - stenosis; bilirubin 2,5 mg/100 ml.

Fig. 7a,b. Cholescintigrams (30 min and 60 min): intensive filling of the
intrahepatic bile ducts (←) and the pre-anastomotic extrahepatic bile duct
(←—); activity in the duodenum (d).

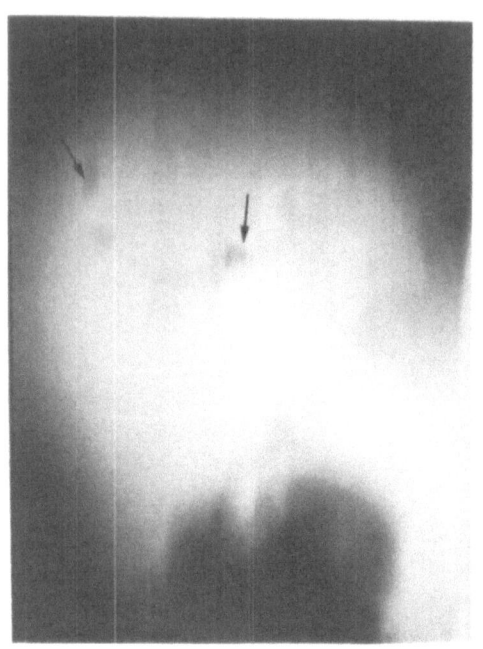 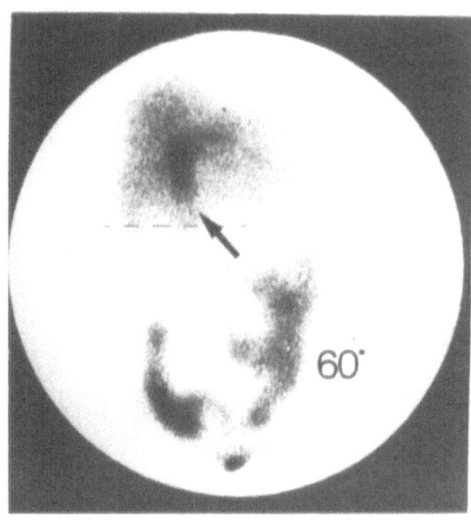

Fig. 8a   Fig. 8b

Fig. 8a. Choledochojejunostomy - stenosis; bilirubin 4 mg/100 ml.

Fig. 8a. Plain abdominal film: slightly widened, air filled intrahepatic ducts
(←).

Fig. 8b. Cholescintigram (60 min): activity break at the anastomosis (◄—) with
activity retention in the pre-anastomotic bile ducts.

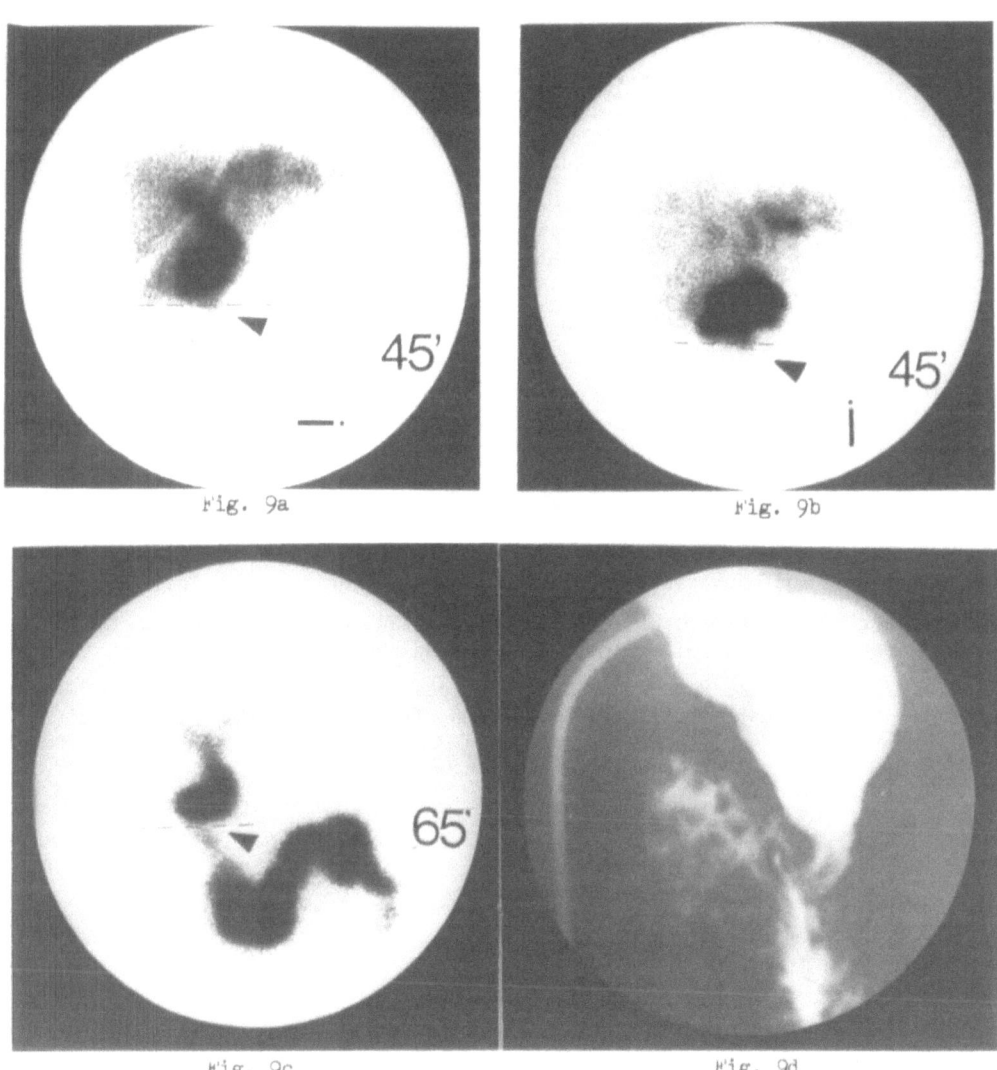

Fig. 9a   Fig. 9b

Fig. 9c   Fig. 9d

Fig. 9c. Choledochojejunostomy - occasional postprandial right upper abdominal discomfort, which disappears after squeezing this area by palpation; bilirubin: normal.

Fig. 9a-c. Cholescintigraphy (45 and 65 min): shifting of the supramesocolic parts of the biliodigestive anastomosis in supine (—-) and up-right (¡) position; emptying after palpating the right upper abdomen; strangulation (◄).

Fig. 9d. Cholangiography shows anatomical situation.

LITERATURE

1. Abou-el-Makarem MM, Millburn P, Smith RL, Williams RT, Differences in the biliary excretion of succinylsulfathiazole. Biochem. J. 105:1269, 1967

2. Baker RJ, Bellen JC, Ronai PM, Technetium-99m-Pyridoxylideneglutamate: a new hepatobiliary radiopharmaceutical. I. Experimental aspects. J. nucl. Med. 16:720, 1975.

3. Kirsch R, Kamisaka K, Fleischner G, Arias IM, Structural and functional studies of ligandin, a major renal organic anion binding protein. J. clin. Invest. 55:1009, 1975.

4. Smith RL, The excretory function of the bile, Chapman and Hall (eds), London, 1973.

5. Maingot R, Operative and postoperative complications. In: Surgery of the gallbladder and bile ducts, Smith R, Sherlock S (eds), London, Butterworths, 1964.

6. Nissen R, Die Vermeidung von Stenoserezidiven nach plastischem Ersatz von Hepaticus und Choledochus. Dtsch. med. Wschr. 84:580, 1959.

7. Reichelt HG, Langenberg G, Löhlein D, Hepato-biliäre Sequenz-Szintigraphie in prä- und postoperativer Oberbauch-Diagnostik. Chirurg 48:583, 1977.

8. Reichelt HG, Die Hepato-biliäre Sequenz Szintigraphie. Entwicklung, Methodik und Empfehlungen für die klinische Anwendung. Röfo 127, 5:427, 1977.

9. Waldram R, Williams R, Calne RY, Bile composition and bile cast formation after transplantation of the liver in man. Transplantation 19:382, 1975.

11. CHOLECYSTITIS

P.H. COX

11.1.INTRODUCTION

Both the acute and chronic forms of cholecystitis may occur in the absence
of gall-stones in up to 10% of all cases but this is obviously to be regarded
as a rarity. In the early stages of the acute disease if the cystic duct is
not blocked by a stone it may be occluded due to the effects of hyperemia and
oedema. In this way bile is prevented from entering or leaving the gall-bladder.
In chronic disease with or without stones the gall-bladder function is impaired
and dependent on the degree to which the cystic duct is damaged, will show impaired filling and emptying.

It is self evident that cholescintigraphy does not provide morphological
information concerning the gall-bladder and bile-ducts and will not visualize
stones. It has however a useful function in demonstrating filling and emptying
of the gall-bladder which makes it possible in turn to demonstrate gall-bladder
malfunction and the presence of obstruction.

A number of authors have proposed the use of Diethyl-Ida cholescintigraphy
as the method of choice for the diagnosis of acute cholecystitis (1,2,3,4,5).
These reports serve to emphasize the fact that the visualization of physiological processes may provide more sensitive diagnostic criteria than does the
visualization of morphological structure.

11.2.Technical requirements for gall-bladder visualization

When Technetium Diethyl-ida is used maximum concentration in the liver is
obtained about 12 minutes post injection. Bile-duct and intestinal activity
can be observed at 15 to 20 minutes post injection and under normal circumstances the gall-bladder will appear on the scintigram between 20 to 40 minutes
post injection. Fig. 1 shows serial scintigrams of a normal subject.

Gall-bladder visualization may not be observed in the normal subject unless
he or she is in the fasting state. Various times of fasting prior to commence-
ment of the study have been recommended but in our experience a period of

4 hours prior to the study gives optimum results. When using reagents other than Diethyl-Ida it should be remembered that the turnover rates may be much slower. Fig. 2 shows serial scintigrams of a normal subject in the non-fasting state to illustrate the non-visualization of the gall-bladder. A repeat study after 4 hours fasting showed normal visualization of the gall-bladder.

When desired gall-bladder emptying can be stimulated by intravenous administration of cholecystokinin (6) or by oral administration of a fatty meal or Sorbitract$^{(R)}$ (7). We have used the latter technique (7) with some success for a number of years. The scanning protocol is outlined in chapter 2. In patients in whom the gall-bladder was visualized but where no intestinal activity was observed at 45 minutes post injection Sorbitract was administered. If then no intestinal activity manifested itself a follow-up scintigram was made 24 hours post injection to confirm delayed intestinal excretion or the presence of complete obstruction.

11.3. Clinical results

An advantage of cholescintigraphy which is emphasized regularly in the literature is that it can be used even in patients with extremely high bilirubin levels with good effect.

Weissmann (1) reported on a series of patients in whom bilirubin levels of up to 8 mg/100 ml were measured. Patency of the cystic duct was demonstrated together with visualization of the gall-bladder in 50 out of 58 cases thus excluding the diagnosis of cholecystitis. Fonseca et al (8) used this method to differentiate between acute cholecystitis and pancreatitis. 13 of 15 patients with acute pancreatitis showed gall-bladder filling thus excluding cholecystitis.

In a study of 113 patients suspected of having cholecystitis 37 were shown to have acute cholecystitis and 39 the chronic form. 38 patients showed normal gall-bladder activity whilst all patients with cholecystitis showed no gall-bladder (9).

Weissmann et al (5) reported on a study of 296 patients with suspected acute cholecystitis. Of these 118 patients with the condition showed non-visualization of the gall-bladder whilst in a further 6 cases it was visible. 171 patients who proved not to have acute cholecystitis showed visualization of the gall-bladder and one other case did not. The accuracy of diagnosis was reported as being 97.6% with a specificity of 99.2% and a sensitivity of 95.2%. An important conclusion drawn by these authors was that the possibility of examining other parameters, as well as gall-bladder visualization, in the same investigation made the diagnosis of other conditions affecting the liver possible whilst excluding cholecystitis.

Shaffer (6) also emphasized the value of evaluating various aspects of Ida-turnover including quantitative measurements. Amongst other things the rate of gall-bladder filling and emptying was recorded and the percentage of activity actually entering the gall-bladder. The relationship between these factors in normal and diseases subjects was examined and changes observed were related to the diseases state.

A typical case of cholecystitis is shown in fig. 3. The relevant case history is given below:

A 58-year old man was admitted with jaundice and fever associated with pain in right upper abdomen.

Laboratory findings:	total bilirubin 58 μmol/l, direct reacting bilirubin 14 μmol/l, alkaline phosphatase 657 mU/ml, SGOT 61 mU/ml, SGPT 117 mU/ml.
Abdominal plain film:	no calcifications in the upper abdomen
Intravenous cholangiography:	stenosed cystic duct
Cholescintigraphy serial scintigraphy (fig. 3-52):	good visualization of the liver without persistent blood-pool activity, visibility of the bileducts with some dilated common bile-duct, no visibility of the gall-bladder, normal intestinal excretion of the radiopharmaceutical
Time activity curves and functional images (fig. 3-53):	normal accumulatory and excretory phases
Conclusion:	suspected gall-bladder pathology
Findings at surgery:	cholecystitis and stones in the gall-bladder.

11.4.Conclusion

Cholescintigraphy appears to be a useful tool to evaluate patients suspected of cholecystitis. In negative cases valuable information can still be obtained by studying the kinetics of Ida-turnover which assists in the identification of the true cause of the symptoms. A problem remains that the technique does not establish the presence of calculi but this can be done by means of other techniques. Small calculi not visible to X-ray or ultrasound have, on the other hand, been demonstrated by showing the effects on bile-flow on the cholescintigram.

166

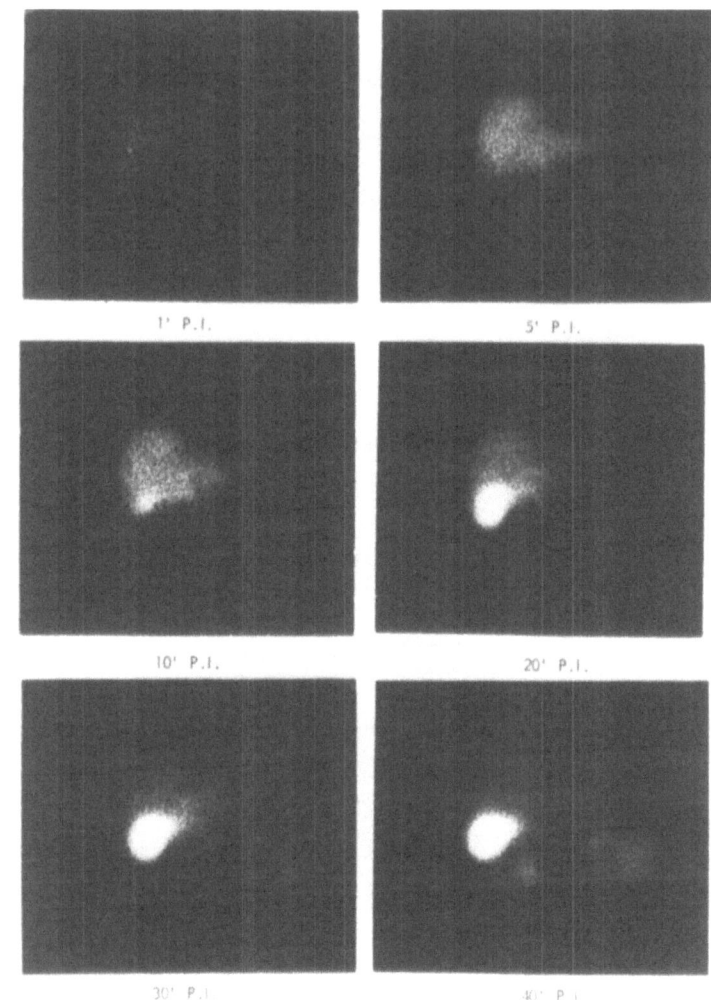

1' P.I.   5' P.I.

10' P.I.   20' P.I.

30' P.I.   40' P.I.

Fig. 1. Normal cholescintigram. Fasting patient.

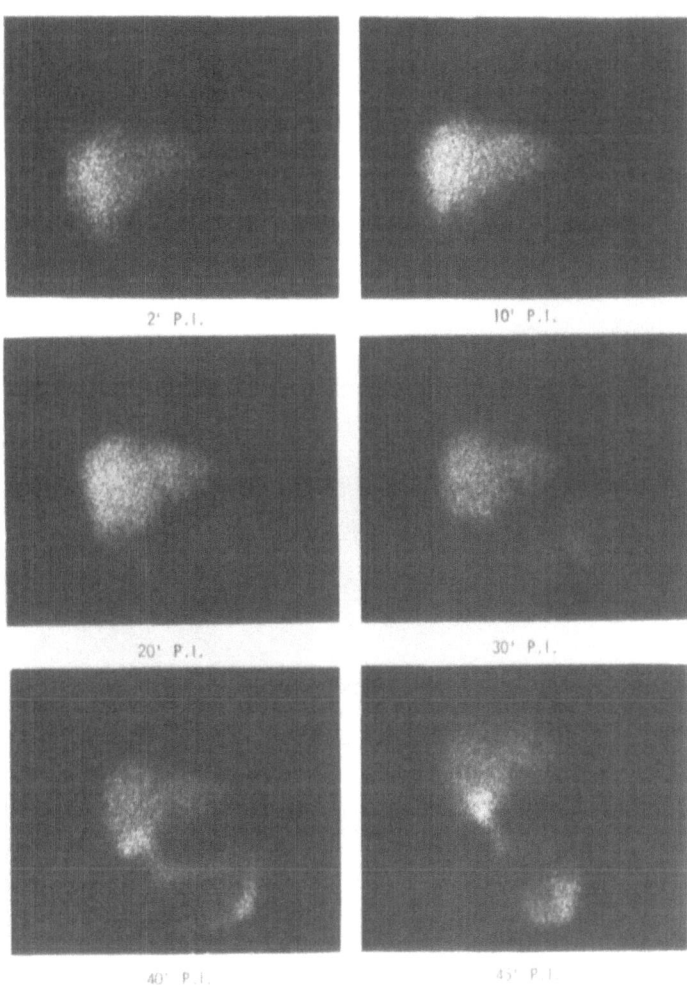

Fig. 2. Normal cholescintigram. Patient non-fasting. Note lack of gall-bladder
activity compared to fig. 1.

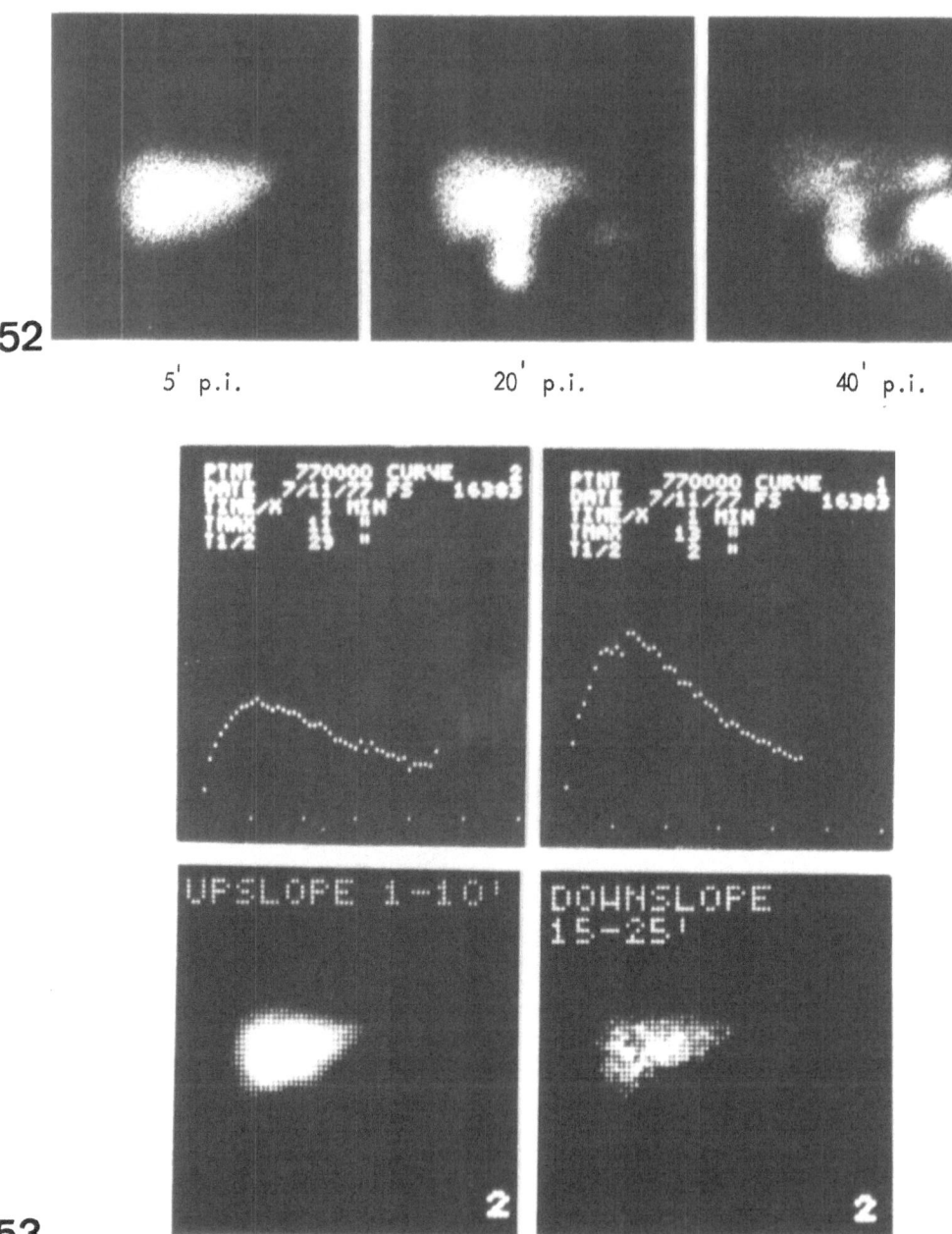

Fig. 3. Cholescintigram of a patient with cholecystitis. See text.

REFERENCES

1. Weissmann HS et al, Rapid and accurate diagnosis of acute cholecystitis with ^{99m}Tc-Hida cholescintigraphy. Amer. J. Roentgenol. 132:523, 1979.

2. Pare P, Shaffer EA, Rosenthall L, Nonvisualization of the gall-bladder by ^{99m}Tc-Hida cholescintigraphy as evidence of cholecystitis. Canad. med. Ass. J. 118:384, 1978.

3. Cheng TH et al, Evaluation of hepatobiliary imaging by radionuclide scintigraphy, ultrasonography and contrast cholangiography. Radiology 133:761, 1979.

4. Weissmann HS et al, Cholescintigraphy, ultrasonography and computerized tomography in the evaluation of biliary tract disorders. Sem. Nucl. Med. 9:22, 1979.

5. Weissmann HS et al, Spectrums of ^{99m}Tc-Ida cholescintigraphic patterns in acute cholecystitis. Radiology 138:167, 1981.

6. Shaffer EA, McOrmond P, Duggan H, Quantitative cholescintigraphy. Assessment of gall-bladder filling and emptying and duodenogastric reflux. Gasteroenterology 79:899, 1980.

7. Tjen HSLM, Cholescintigraphy Ph.D. Thesis, University of Utrecht, The Netherlands (in English), 1979.

8. Fonseca C et al, ^{99m}Tc-ida imaging in the differential diagnosis of acute cholecystitis and acute pancreatitis. Radiology 130:525, 1979.

9. Fonseca C et al, Tc-ida imaging in the evaluation of cholecystitis. Clin. nucl. Med. 3:437, 1978.

12. QUANTITATIVE STUDIES OF HEPATOBILIARY TRANSPORT

P.H. COX

12.1. INTRODUCTION

By observing the changing distribution patterns on serial scintigrams the uptake of Ida-derivatives from the blood stream into the hepatocytes and their subsequent secretion into the gall-bladder and intestine can be followed. Deviations from the normal pattern can be used to identify obstructive disease, gall-bladder abnormalities and hepatocyte malfunction.

The overall accuracy of serial scintigraphy lies in the region of 70%. In the detection of obstructive disease this approaches 100% but in the case of functional disease small foci or general diffuse parenchymal disease may not be observed by visual assessment alone. The mass of normally functioning tissue may mask the presence of disease. Quantification of the study using gamma camera on line computer combinations can significantly improve the rate of detection of pathology in such cases.

It is not the intention to go into the technical details of such techniques here since the relevant information is already available in the literature (1, 2,3,4), but to outline some of the procedures which have been used to evaluate Ida-turnover in the liver.

12.2. Functional indices

Probably the simplest technique which has been used to date is the calculation of functional indices. Count rates are recorded in selected regions of interest in the liver at fixed times post injection and ratios are computed. Using this technique Pors Nielsen et al (5) calculated a retention index, the activity at the time of maximum concentration in the liver divided into the activity in the same region 30 minutes post injection. An index of hepatic uptake was calculated by dividy the activity measured in the right liver lobe at 5 minutes post injection by the activity measured over the abdominal aorta at the same time.

The excretory capacity of the liver was estimated by calculating a retention index which was defined as the ratio between the measured activity in the right liver lobe at maximum concentrations and that measured 30 minutes post injection.

The results obtained using these functional indices were considered to provide useful information when combined with serial scintigraphy and time activity curves.

12.3. Time activity curves

Every scintigram represents the biological distribution of the reagent, in the organ to be studied, at a moment in time. As such it reflects physiology rather than morphology although morphological information can be deduced.

If however the changes in activity concentrations with respect to time are recorded time activity distribution curves can be plotted for selected regions of interest. Probably the best known example of this is the renogram.

In the past hepatocyte function has been assessed by recording time activity curves for the hepatic uptake of rectally administered Pertechnetate, the so called hepatogram (6).

The measurement of time activity curves for selected regions of interest over the liver using Ida-derivatives and Diethyl-Ida in particular, has proved to be of considerable diagnostic value (5,7,8). Liver time activity curves either for the whole liver or for regions of interest coupled with a heart blood activity curve can be used to provide a number of quantitative measurements of diagnostic value such as the $T\frac{1}{2}$ blood clearance, T max hepatic uptake, $T\frac{1}{2}$ liver clearance and liver transit time. Time activity curves from regions of interest however suffer from the clear disadvantage that they do not provide pure data concerning hepatocyte turnover but also register effects due to blood-pool activity, bile duct build up and transport. Hence small foci of disease may be missed due to the masking effect of surrounding normal hepatocyte activity and it is impossible to differentiate between diffuse intra hepatic and extra hepatic obstruction. Hence whilst the use of time activity curves combined with serial scintigraphy improves the diagnostic accuracy of the method to above 80% more refined techniques are necessary in order to obtain maximum results.

12.4. Compartmental analysis

The application of the analysis of reagent distribution, in differing components of the liver, in relation to time on the basis of a multicompartment model is not new (9) and has been applied to Ida-derivatives (10). Is has however been pointed out that this approach suffers from a number of pitfalls (11).

In the first place the use of a compartment model assumes that the activity in each compartment (blood, hepatocytes and bile) can be monitored separately which is not the case. The liver activity measured in any one region of interest contains all components and the biliary component is even more complicated since it includes both capillaries, collecting ducts and main bile trunks which have different kinetics.

It has been shown (5,11) that time activity curves generated from peripheral regions of the liver, where the bile-duct contribution is minimal do fit a simple compartment model quite well. However the restriction of regions of interest to peripheral areas is only applicable to the diagnosis of generally disseminated disease and therefore inherently has a limited practical value.

The use of a large number of small regions of interest to provide data for compartmental analysis or time activity curves minimizes all of these problems to some extent but is time consuming and difficult to interpret.

12.5. Functional imaging

An alternative approach which is more sophisticated and elegant is functional imaging. This technique makes optimum use of the gamma camera computer system. A quantitative assessment of the kinetics of the bio distribution of the reagent is made which is presented in the form of a static image.

The idea of functional images was first muted by Kaihara in 1969 (12) and has been explored by a number of workers. A recent general review of the technique was made by Crespo-Diez (13). Van Rijk (14) first applied the technique to liver function studies using a method developed by De Graaf (3,11). A modified version of this method was used by Cox and Tjen to evaluate Diethyl-ida kinetics with excellent results (7,15,16,17).

With the functional imaging as applied to Diethyl-Ida studies the rate of change of Diethyl-Ida concentration at each point in the 64 x 64 computer matrix covering the field of view of the gamma camera is measured. A time activity curve is generated for each point and the slopes (rate of change) of the accumulation and excretory phases are calculated. For any given phase the rate of change is assessed and assigned to a category in a gray scale which is then reproduced as an image in which the brightness of each picture element (pixel) reflects the rate of change of activity: the more rapid the rate of change the brighter the pixel. Each pixel corresponds to a very small region of liver tissue so that small diseases foci or diffusely disseminated disease are more readily detected.

For each study two functional images are generated, i.e. accumulatory phase (upslope) and excretory phase (downslope), for the Diethyl-Ida turnover. In a normal subject a homogenous image is obtained whilst in the diseased state an inhomogenous image will be observed. It is however important to prepare time activity curves for both the right and left lobes as well because in the event of a uniformly distributed parenchymal disease a homogenous functional image may be obtained.

Fig. 1 shows the functional images obtained from a normal subject. The upper left is the accumulatory image and middle the excretory phase. The right hand image is an accumulatory image prepared during the excretory phase only bile-ducts and gall-bladder are visible. The hepatocytes are not accumulating activity in this phase, thus are not visible. The use of this method has been discussed further in chapter 7.

Fig. 2 shows serial scintigrams, functional images and time activity curves of a patient with metastatic disease of the right liver lobe. The left lobe shows normal Diethyl-Ida uptake in the serial scintigram (top) and a normal time activity curve (bottom right) but the downslope functional image (middle right) shows a disturbed function. The presence of diffuse metastases was later confirmed. This example serves to show how it is desirable to make both curves and functional images as well as serial scintigrams.

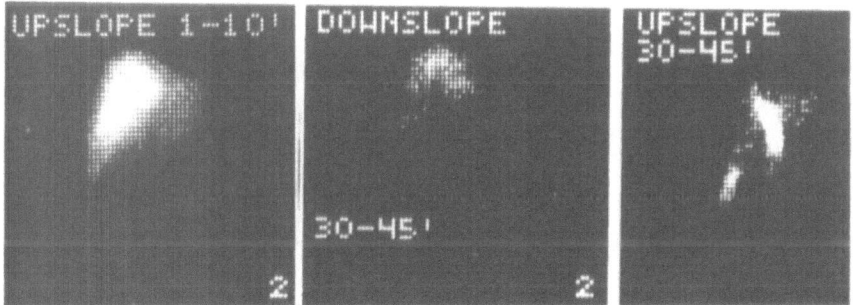

Fig. 1. Functional images of a normal individual - see text.

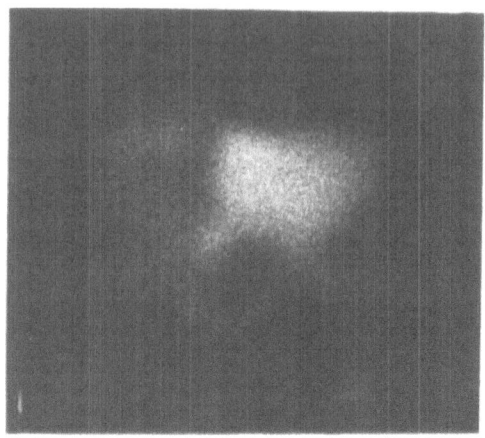

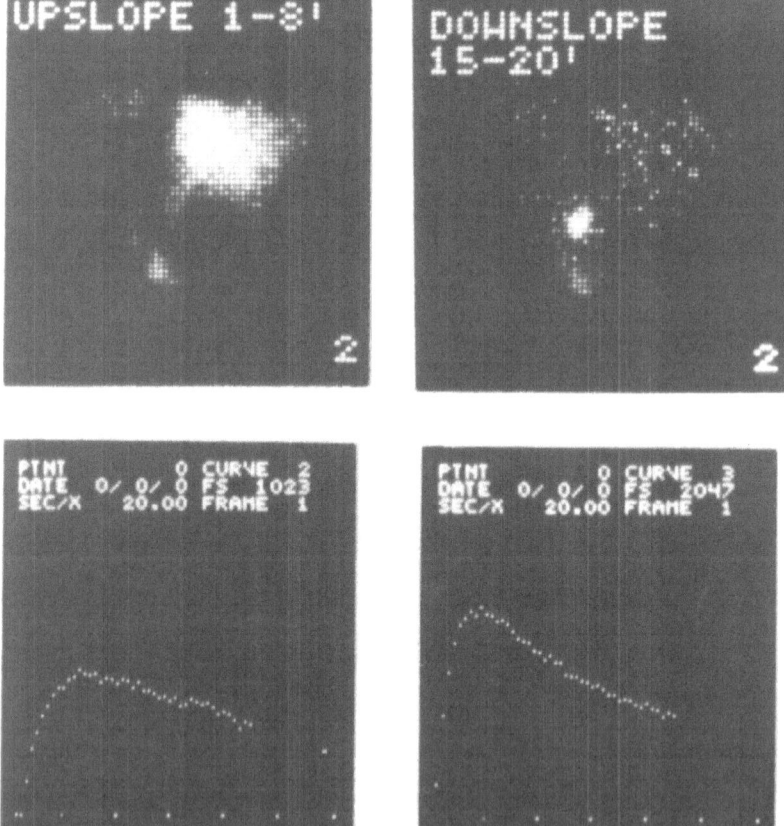

Fig. 2. Patient with metastatic disease. Top: serial scintigram. Middle: left and right up- and downslope functional images. Bottom: time activity curves for the right and left lobes respectively - see text.

REFERENCES

1. Kenny PJ, Smith EM, Quantitative organ visualisation. University Press of Miami, 1971.

2. Hoekstra A, Instrumentation in Nuclear Medicine. In: Proceedings of a Symposium on Nuclear Medicine, Ephraim KH, Yoe OH (eds), University of Utrecht, 1975.

3. De Graaf CN, Developments in information processing in Nuclear Medicine. In: Proceedings of a Symposium on Nuclear Medicine, Ephraim KH, Yoe OH (eds), University of Utrecht, 1975.

4. De Graaf CN, Information processing in the evaluation of ^{99m}Tc-ida studies. In: Progress in Radiopharmacology, Vol. I. Cox PH (ed), Amsterdam, Elsevier/North-Holland Biomedical Press, 1979.

5. Pors Nielsen S et al, Hepatobiliary scintigraphy and hepatography with ^{99m}Tc-diethyl ida in obstructive jaundice. J. nucl. Med. 19:452, 1978.

6. Van Bochove WM, Hepatografie met ^{99m} Tc pertechnetate. Ph.D. Thesis, University of Amsterdam, 1970.

7. Tjen HSLM, Cholescintigraphy Ph.D. Thesis, University of Utrecht (in English), 1979.

8. Biersack HJ, Mahlstedt J, Hepatobiliary scintigraphy by means of Ida derivatives. Darmstadt, G-I-T-/E Giebler, 1978.

9. Quarfordt SH et al, Compartmental analysis of sulphobromophtalein transport in normal patients and patients with hepatic dysfunction. Gastroenterology 60:246, 1971.

10. Venot A et al, Improvement of dynamic cholescintigraphy through mathematical modelling of ^{99m}Tc diethyl ida pharmacokinetics. Ann. Insorm. 1978.

11. De Graaf CN, Information processing in the evaluation of ^{99m}Tc-ida studies. In: Progress in Radiopharmacology. Vol. I. Cox PH (ed), Amsterdam, Elsevier/North-Holland Biomedical Press, 1979,

12. Kaihara S et al, Construction of a functional image from regional rate constants. J. nucl. Med. 10:347, 1969.

13. Crespo-Diez A et al, Functional scintigraphy. In: Nuklearmedizin - Clinical value of Nuclear Medicine Methods. Schmidt HAE, Ortiz Berrocal J (eds), Stuttgart, Schattauer, 1979.

14. Van Rijk PP, Purifications labelling and clinical applicability of radioactive asialo orosomucoid. Ph.D. Thesis, University of Utrecht, 1977.

15. Cox PH et al, Technetium ^{99m} diethylacetamilidoiminodiacetate combined with functional imaging for the study of hepatocyte function. In: Nuklearmedizin - state of the art and future. Schmidt HAE, Woldring MG (eds), Stuttgart, Schattauer, 1978.

16. Cox PH, The clinical application of functional imaging. In: Hepatobiliary scintigraphy by means of ida derivatives. Biersack HJ, Mahlstedt J (eds), Darmstadt, G-I-T-/E Giebler, 1978.

17. Tjen HSLM, Cox PH, The use of ^{99m}Tc diethylida combined with functional imaging for the differentiation of obstructive and functional jaundice. In: Nuklearmedizin. Schmidt HAE, Ortiz Berrocal J (eds), Stuttgart, Schattauer, 1979.

13. CHOLESCINTIGRAPHY: ITS DIAGNOSTIC SIGNIFICANCE IN COMPARISON TO
SONOGRAPHY, CT, X-RAY AND LABORATORY TESTS

H.J. BIERSACK

13.1. INTRODUCTION

There are only a few areas in internal medicine other than the diseases of
liver and biliary tract in which such rapid improvements in diagnosis have been
achieved. New procedures such as endoscopic retrogade cholangio-pancreatico-
graphy (ERCP), percutaneous transhepatic cholangiography (PTC), computed tomography (CT), and ultrasonography (US) have gained importance beside the well
known diagnostic tools like intravenous cholangiography (IVC) and laboratory
tests. At the end of 1971 (1) the spectrum of non-invasive methods was
increased by the addition of cholescintigraphy with pyridoxylidene glutamate
(1) and Ida-derivatives (2). The latter have proved to be the reagents of
choice (3).

The diagnostic procedures mentioned here are of particular importance
since the anamnesis, clinical findings, and laboratory tests are often helpful
in the differential diagnosis of ultra- and extrahepatic cholestasis. This
question, however, should be answered in the case of cholestasis during the
first 3 weeks after onset of the disease. The frequency and severity of postoperative complications increase if the performance of necessary surgical intervention is delayed. Duration of the jaundice for more than 2 weeks may cause
irreversible damage to the liver parenchyma. For example, postoperative mortality is increasing from 4 to 19% in cholelithiasis and from 29 to 58% in
malignant obstructive jaundice when the jaundice is lasting longer than 3
weeks (4). These facts demonstrate the importance of non-invasive diagnostic
procedures as screening methods in the differential diagnosis of cholestasis.
In the following subchapters the results of cholescintigraphy have been compared to those of the previously mentioned procedures. The purpose of this
comparison is to evaluate the diagnostic significance of cholescintigraphy and
to make a recommendation for its application.

13.2.Cholescintigraphy and liver scintigraphy with colloids

The area of the gall-bladder even in normal subjects can cause "cold lesions" in liver scintigraphy (5,6) which is particularly the case with intra-hepatic gall-bladders (6). In such cases cholescintigraphy may be helpful to clarify the findings by verifying the filling of this area by the gall-bladder. In this way combination of colloid and Ida-scintigraphy can help to avoid false-positive results. Fig. 1 shows such an example: the colloid liver-scan (fig. 1a) reveals a filling defect in the caudal portion of the right lobe. Cholescintigraphy (fig. 1b), however, reveals that the defect is an artefact caused by the gall-bladder.

If even in normal controls these diagnostic artefacts may appear, the problems are increased when obstructive jaundice is present. This is due to defects - particularly in the hilar region - which are caused by the dilated bile-ducts (7,8,9). Histopathological findings revealed that obstructive jaundice with the respective defects led to the misdiagnosis (liver metastases" in some cases (9).

The exclusion of an assumed accessory spleen after splenectomy is possible by the demonstration of functioning liver tissue in the former splenic bed when both Ida and colloid-scintigraphy are performed (5). Fig. 2 shows a respective case with the accumulation of Sulphur colloid (fig. 2a) as well as Ida (fig. 2b). The combination of colloid and Ida-scintigraphy is, however, of particular importance in longlasting complete obstructive jaundice when accumu-lation of Ida in the liver parenchyma no longer occurs. In many cases with complete obstruction of the bile-ducts a normal colloid liver-scan may be seen whilst a Ida-scintigraphy no longer provides diagnostic information because the tracer is totally excreted through the kidneys. Hence by the different results of colloid-scintigraphy (normal uptake of the colloid) and Ida-scinti-graphy (complete renal retention), the definite diagnosis of obstructive jaundice can be made. Fig. 3 shows such a case with normal colloid-scan (fig. 3a) and no Ida accumulation in liver and intestines up to 24 hours (fig. 3b). In severe parenchymal damage on the contrary colloid accumulation is greatly re-duced in the liver (fig. 4a) whilst Ida-scintigraphy shows a good visualization of the gall-bladder and gastro intestinal-tract (fig. 4b).

To sum up in conclusion, it can be stated that cholescintigraphy should in any event be combined with colloid liver-scintigraphy in order to achieve the highest diagnostic accuracy. In the differential diagnosis of longblasting obstructive jaundice, liver-scintigraphy with Tc^{99m} labeled colloids is of

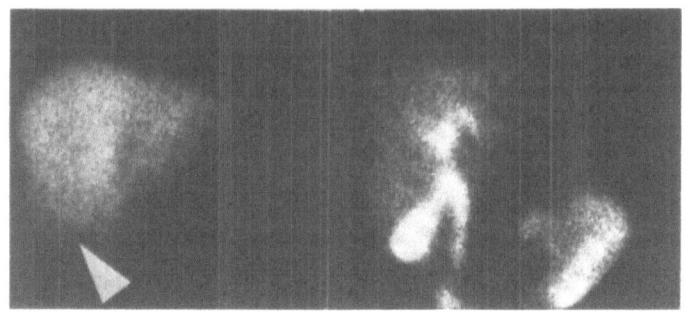

Fig. 1a   Fig. 1b

Fig. 1. Assumed filling defect in the right liver lobe
a) Liver-scan with Tc^{99n} Sulphur colloid: assumed filling defect in the caudal portion of the right liver lobe.
b) Scintigraphy with Tc^{99m}-Ida: the defect is filled up by the tracer thus being identified as gall-bladder bed.

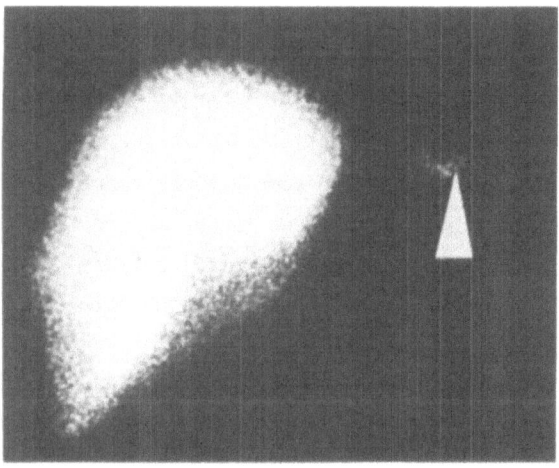

Fig. 2a

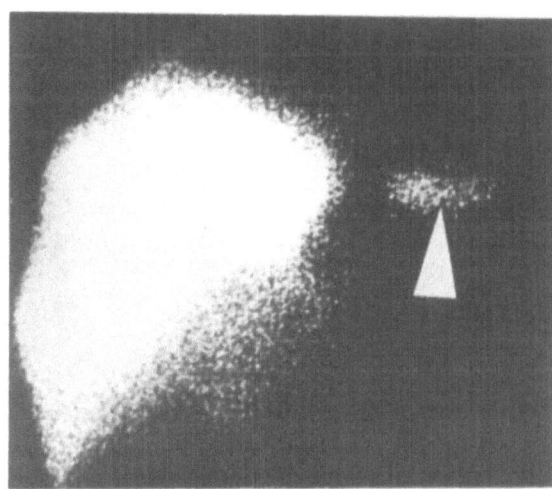

Fig. 2b

Fig. 2. Assumed acessory spleen: tissue in the area of the assumed acessory spleen is taking up Sulphur colloid (a) <u>and</u> Ida (b) thus ruling out splenic tissue.

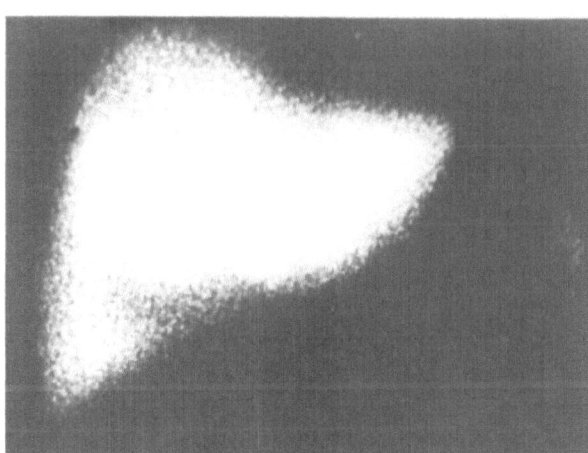

Fig. 3a

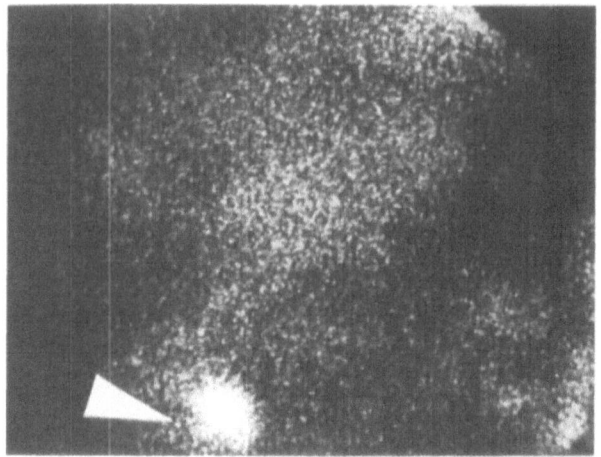

Fig. 3b

Fig. 3. Obstructive jaundice: regular uptake of Sulphur colloid in the liver (a) complete <u>renal</u> excretion (⟶) of Ida with no accumulation of the tracer in the liver tissue (b).

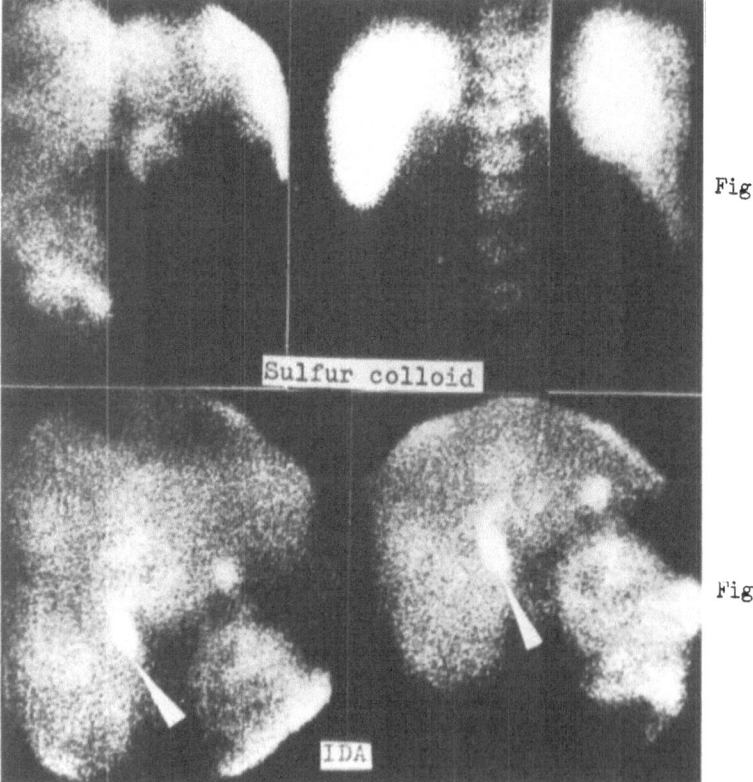

Sulfur colloid

Fig. 4a

Fig. 4b

IDA

Fig. 4. Liver cirrhosis: typical scintigraphic picture of liver cirrhosis (a, Sulphur colloid); good visualization of gall-bladder and GI tract by Ida-scintigraphy (b).

essential value.

13.3.Cholescintigraphy and ultrasonography

In the differential diagnosis of jaundice both cholescintigraphy and ultrasound offer superior possibilities. The basis of the sonographic evaluation is
the visualization of normal or dilated bile-ducts. The direct diagnosis of
parenchymal damage by ultrasound is difficult (10). The investigations of
Dewbury et al (19) have shown that the diagnosis of liver cirrhosis by echo
patterns is only possible in 65% of the cases studied. Thirty-five percent of
these patients had normal echo pattern and no bright (cirrhosis-specific)
pattern. In 50% of patients with cirrhosis and normal echo pattern, however,
diagnosis of parenchymal damage could be confirmed by the demonstration of
hepato- and/or splenomegaly, ascites, and enlargement of the portal vein.
Heilmann (11) found 21% false negatives in a series of more than 500 patients
with parenchymal damage when the spleen was evaluated in addition to the liver
echogram. According to Albertson and Leopold (12) fibrotic replacement only is
to be seen late in the course of the disease so that the typical bright echos
are not present in the early stages of liver cirrhosis. Diagnostic problems
occur in the evaluation of regenerative nodules which have to be differentiated
from hepatoma (12).

With regard to the accuracy of ultrasonography in the diagnosis of parenchymal damage (about 70-80%) it can be stated that cholescintigraphy (over 90%
correct positives) is superior. This fact, however, should be considered
bearing in mind that the diagnosis of diffuse liver disease is a primarily
domain where laboratory tests are used. Only if jaundice is present do these
tests lose their value particularly when evaluating the differential diagnosis
of jaundice.

Fig. 5 shows the complementary nature of the results in a patient with
jaundice liver cirrhosis: fig. 5a presents the cholescintigraphic result with
reduced activity accumulation in the liver but good excretion of the bile into
the intestines. Fig. 5b gives an example of the typical bright echo patterns.

When considering the detection of dilated bile-ducts in obstructive jaundice
ultrasound shows a high accuracy (12,13,14,15). However, the sonographic image
in dilatation of the biliary system (multiple dense echos in the liver) may be
misinterpreted in some cases (12). In most cases the diagnosis is made possible
by visualization of prominent tubular and branching structures (12). Furthermore,
a confusion between a dilated common bile-duct and the portal vein can be

avoided by considering the topography (common bile-duct descends posteriorly from the gall-bladder and cystic-duct) (12). According to Dewburry et al (16) and Rettenmeier et al (13) the diagnostic accuracy in obstructive jaundice is about 97%. In 58% of these patients aetiologic diagnosis can also be made (16). It should be mentioned that the common bile-duct is considered to be dilated if its diameter is more than 8 to 14 mm (15,16) when estimated by sonography.

With regard to the results of cholescintigraphy it can be stated that this method allows the evaluation of the cause of a jaundice in over 90% of cases by the prescence or absence of excretion of the bile into the intestines (17,18), but visualization of the bile-ducts is only possible in incomplete obstruction (3). Untill now there have been numerous papers published dealing with the comparison between cholescintigraphic and ultrasound studies in obstructive jaundice (18,19,20,21,22,23). Klingensmith et al (20) observed a superiority of cholescintigraphy when compared to ultrasound. A combination of both methods, however, improved the specificity without loss of sensitivity. These results are confirmed by Pauwels et al (18). Ryan et al (19) recommend ultrasound as the first step in the evaluation of jaundice. If this procedure demonstrates dila-ted bile-ducts cholescintigraphy is not necessary. If normal bile-ducts are present cholescintigraphy should be performed in order to differentiate between incomplete obstruction and parenchymal jaundice. In our opinion this diagnostic procedure cannot be recommended unrestrictedly because in many cases dilated bile-ducts are present despite of normal bile excretion. Fig. 6 shows the ultra-sound and the cholescintigraphic results in such a patient: ultrasound demon-strates dilated bile-ducts (fig. 6a.) while cholescintigraphy shows stenosis of the papilla but normal bile excretion (fig. 6b). Fig. 7 presents the "normal findings" in obstructive jaundice with dilated bile-ducts (fig. 7a) visible to ultrasound but no excretion of the reagent into the gastro-intestinal tract during Ida-scintigraphy up to 24 hours post injection(fig. 7). However, chole-scintigraphy has gained high importance in the evaluation of acute obstructive jaundice without dilated bile-ducts. Some cases of obstruction without ductal dilatation have been described by Weismann et al (24). These authors have demonstrated cholescintigraphy to be a sensitive and reliable method for detect-ing the functional abnormality of obstruction before the morphologic changes due to dilatation is seen in ultrasonography and even before the liver function tests are abnormal (24). Of the 20 patients in this group who had both ultrasound and cholescintigraphy, 14 (is 70%) showed the common bile-duct to have normal dimen-sions on ultrasound. Fig. 4 shows the respective results in a patient early after

onset of obstruction with absent bile excretion into the intestines (fig. 8a)
but normal bile-ducts in the ultrasound study (fig. 8b).

Diseases of the gall-bladder are nowadays a domain of ultrasound (25).
Safe diagnosis of the localization of the gall-bladder as well as evaluation of
its configuration and wall is possible by this method. With regard to the diagnostic accuracy, it is at least equal to the conventional X-ray procedures such
as IVC or infusion cholecystography (26,27,28,29). New results published by
Cooperberg and Burhenne (30) have led to the opinion that IVC can be replaced
by ultrasound. The sonographic picture of inflammation of the gall-bladder
consists of thickening and double contour of the gall-bladder wall. In acute
cholecystitis cholescintigraphic diagnosis is made by the absence of gall-
bladder visualization because of cystic-duct obstruction (31,32). The diagnostic
accuracy in this disease is about 90% using Ida-derivatives if gall-bladder (non)
visualization on delayed views up to 4 hours was considered (33). Thus, cholescintigraphy has a higher sensitivity than ultrasound. In chronic cholecystitis,
however, gall-bladder visualization can be observed in some cases which makes
differential diagnosis impossible (34). Considering the fact that the gall-
bladder may be visualized up to 2 hours post injection in normal controls with
"excretion type" bile excretion (35), the differential diagnosis of gall-bladder
diseases will be even more complicated. Fig. 9 shows a synopsis of the results
in cholecystitis: cholescintigraphic diagnosis is made by the nonvisualization
of the gall-bladder (fig. 9a), sonography shows the thickening of the gall-
bladder wall (fig. 9b).

In the diagnosis of concretions ultrasound cannot be replaced by cholescintigraphy. The sonographic diagnosis of concretions is based on the fact
that gall-stones are producing strong echos and absorption of the ultrasonic
beam results in accoustic shadows distally. Concretions with a diameter less
than 2 mm cannot be visualized by ultrasound (12). Braun (36) was able to
demonstrate an accuracy of about 99% concerning the diagnosis of gall-stones by
ultrasound. Sonography, therefore, is the diagnostic procedure of choice in
cholelithiasis. Cholescintigraphy is not indicative of gall-bladder concretions.

Intrahepatic calculi are also a domain of ultrasound. Sonographic diagnosis
is again made by the proof of amplification and consecutive absorption of echos.
Cholescintigraphy exhibits obstruction of the bile-flow in the respective intrahepatic bile-ducts (37). If sonography is not sucessfully performed, cholescintigraphy may be used for this purpose.

On the basis of this information can be stated that the comparison of the

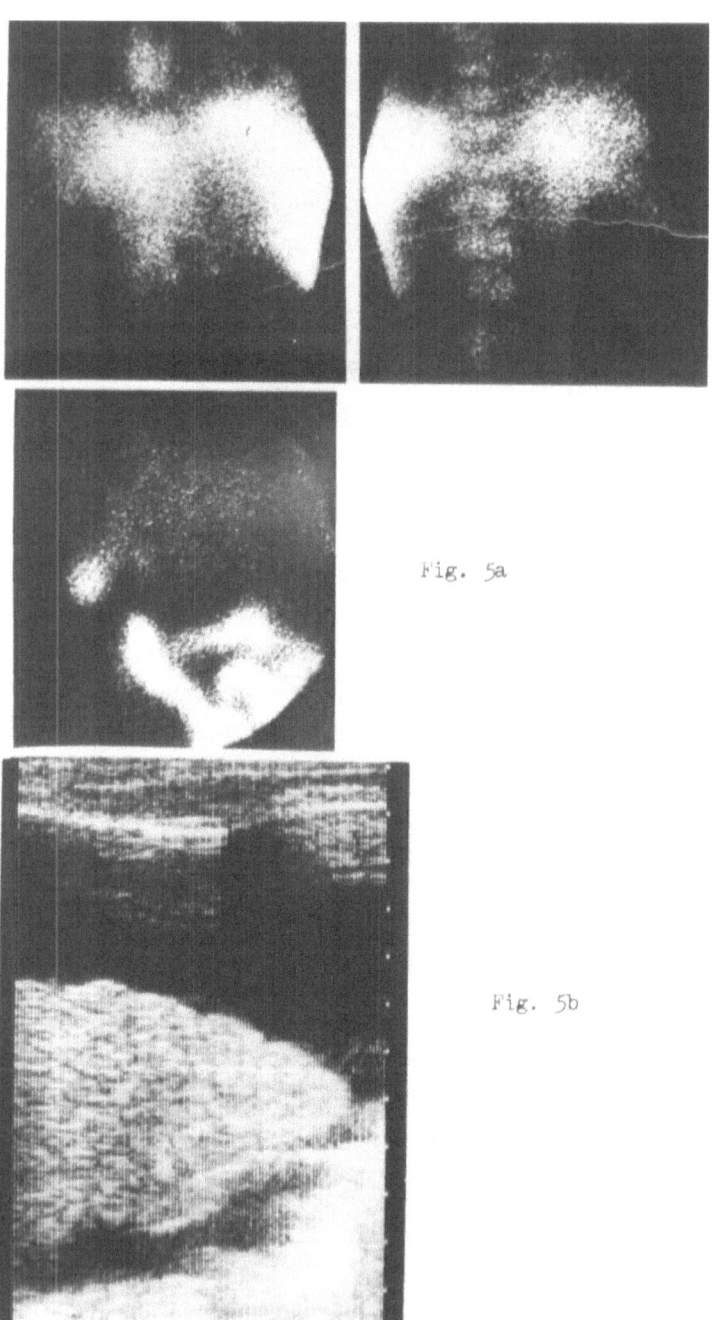

Fig. 5a

Fig. 5b

Fig.5 . Liver cirrhosis:
a) Sulphur colloid liver-scan (left, middle) and Ida-scintigraphy (right):
good visualization of bile into the intestines.
b) US with typical "bright echo pattern" and ascites.

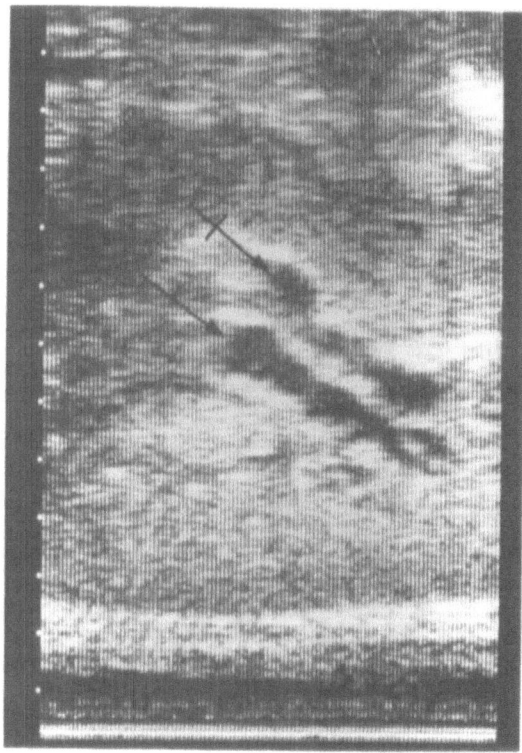

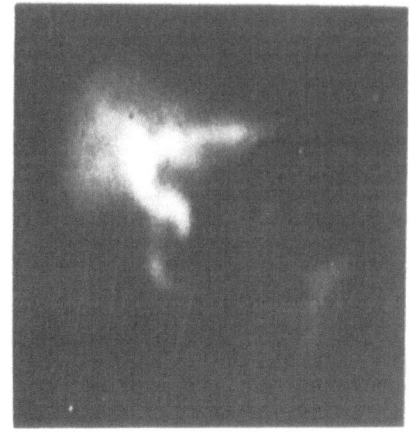

Fig. 6b

Fig. 6a

Fig. 6 . Stenosis of the papilla:
a) US: moderately dilated bile ducts
b) Ida-scintigraphy: stenosis of the papilla but regular bile excretion.

186

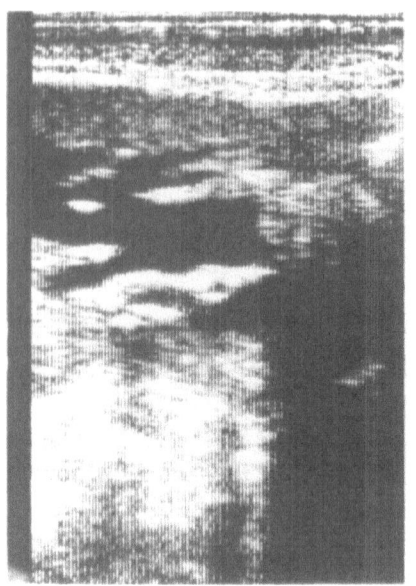

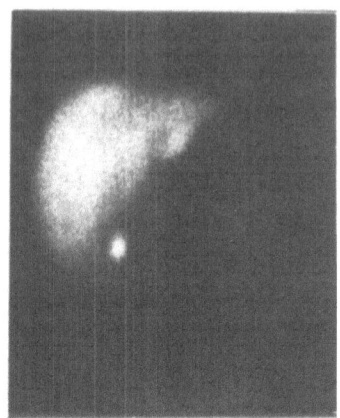

Fig. 7b

Fig. 7a

Fig. 7. Complete obstructive jaundice:
a) US: dilated bile ducts.
b) Ida-scintigraphy: no intestinal bile excretion

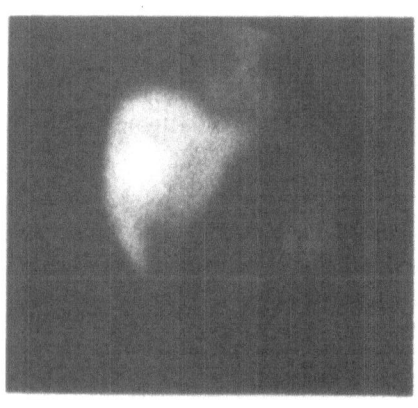

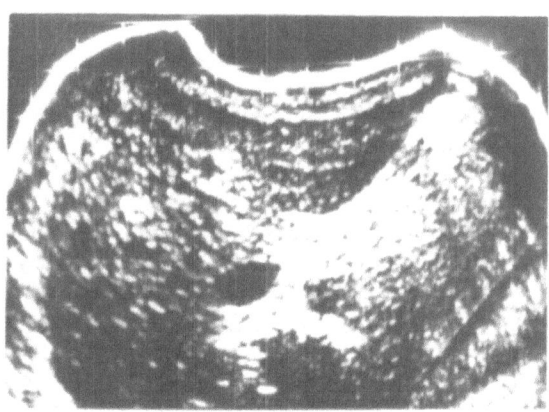

Fig. 8a

Fig. 8b

Fig. 8 . Obstructive jaundice early after onset of the disease:
a) Ida-scintigraphy: good accumulation of the tracer in the liver but no bile
discharge into the intestines.
b) US: normal width of the bile ducts.

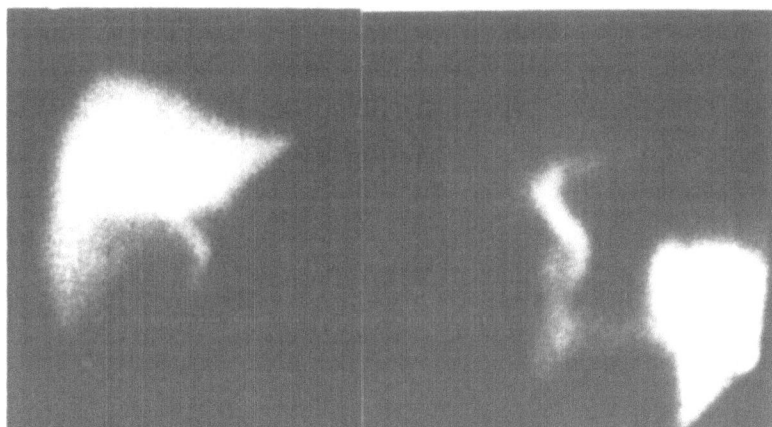

Fig. 9a

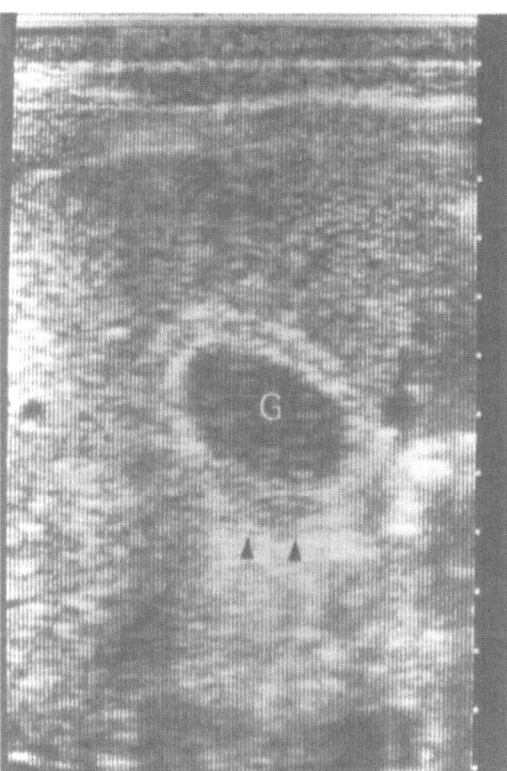

Fig. 9b

Fig. 9. Cholecystitis:
a) Ida-scintigraphy: regular discharge of the bile into the GI tract but non-visualization of the gall-bladder.
b) US: thickening of the gall-bladder wall.

two methods shows up two main indications for cholescintigraphy:

1. It is a sensitive and reliable method for detecting biliary obstruction before the morphologic change of dilation of the biliary system is seen.

2. Cholescintigraphy can be considered as the method of choice in the differential diagnosis of acute pancreatitis and acute cholecystitis with a sensitivity and specificity of about 99% (33).

If dilation of the bile-ducts is already present in obstructive jaundice cholescintigraphy and ultrasound yield a similar diagnostic accuracy (over 90%). Ultrasound, however, offers the advantage of aetiologic diagnosis in about 60% of cases. In biliary diseases without jaundice but with dilated bile-ducts cholescintigraphy is able to answer the question whether relevant obstruction to bile-flow is actually present or not. In the case of parenchymal damage cholescintigraphy is superior to ultrasound by the demonstration of normal bile-flow to the intestines as well as in the detection of diffuse liver disease. The diagnosis of chronic gall-bladder disease can only be made using sonography.

13.4. Cholescintigraphy and computed tomography (CT)

CT offers - like sonography - the possibility of visualizing dilated bile-ducts in obstructive jaundice. The application of contrast media leads to a better delineation of the biliary system. Diagnosis of concretions is easily made due to their high density (39).

Diagnosis of diffuse parenchymal damage usually causes problems: according to Scherer et al (39) the diagnostic accuracy in only about 20% which is confirmed by the paper of Levitt et al (40). Cholescintigraphy, however, offers the possibility of the early detection of impaired reagent kinetics in diffuse liver disease.

CT investigations by Scherer et al (39) concerning the differential diagnosis of jaundice yielded the following results: the diagnostic accuracy in parenchymal jaundice was about 100%, in obstructive jaundice, however, the accuracy was only about 77% (39) compared with over 90% correct positive cholescintigraphic results (3,18). Fig.10 shows a synopsis of CT and cholescintigraphic results in a patient with obstructive jaundice: CT (fig. 10a) visualized dilated bile-ducts, the cholescintigraphic image (fig. 10b) shows the pathognomonic pattern of biliary obstruction with no accumulation of activity within the intestines up to 24 hours.

Until now, there have been numerous published papers comparing the results of colloid scintigraphy with those of CT (41,42,43,44,45), an

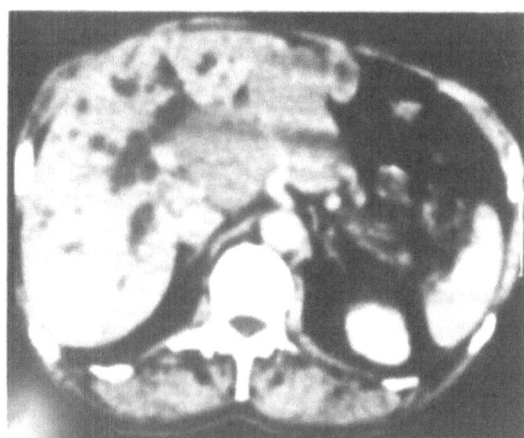

Fig. 10a

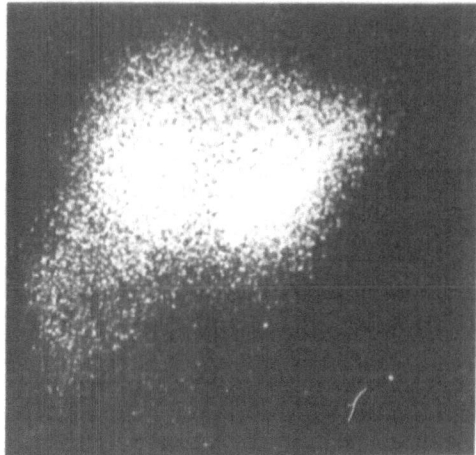

Fig. 10b

Fig.10. Obstructive jaundice:
a) CT: dilated bile ducts because of hilar lymphomas.
b) Ida-scintigraphy (24 hours post injection): no bile discharge into the intestines.

evaluation of CT and cholescintigraphy is only mentioned in a paper presented by Weissmann et al (32). The authors stress the point that cholescintigraphy is of high value in the differential diagnosis of jaundice. CT of the liver is in our opinion most useful in the aetiologic diagnosis of the cause of obstruction, e.g. cholelithiasis, tumour of the papilla, and pancreas carcinoma.

To summarize these considerations it can be stated that in the differential diagnosis of jaundice cholescintigraphic.investigation should be performed prior to CT. If obstruction of the bile-ducts is present the aetiologic should be evaluated with CT. Regarding diseases of the gall-bladder CT results can be compared with those of sonography: concretions as well as thickened gall-bladder wall can be visualized by both methods. CT is, therefore, superior to chole-scintigraphy in gall-bladder diseases.

13.5. Cholescintigraphy and intravenous cholangiography (IVC)

The X-ray diagnosis of the biliary tract should in any event be started with a plain film of the abdomen which allows the visualization of small calculi. Furthermore, this procedure is suited to give information on the probable presence of porcelain gall-bladder or chalk milk bile.

This investigation should be followed by intravenous cholangio-cholecysto-graphy which visualizes the gall-bladder and the biliary tract after orally or intravenously administered contrast media. With high bilirubin levels (above 2 mg%) IVC should be performed as long time infusion cholangiography. The diagnostic accuracy is strongly limited above bilirubin levels of 2 mg. If the bilirubin is above 4 mg% diagnosis is possible in only some rare cases. As the common bile-duct is only visualized in about 10% of the cases (46) X-ray tomography has to be done. This method leads to an improvement of IVC so that the common bile-duct can be evaluated in about 80% (47) In every case where contrast media are used the risk of incompatibility reactions should be taken into consideration. According to Stauch et al (48) in about 20 to 30% of these reactions can be observed. Side reactions which need treatment occur in at least 4% (48). Elevations of transaminases in diffuse parenchymal damage were reported after injection of Ioglycamide (49). These reactions, however, were not present after administration of Iodooxamine acid (49). Winckler et al (50) reported some cases with histopathological findings of focal liver necrosis after infusion cholangiography. Furthermore, exacerbation and manifestation of hyperthyreoidism should be considered in connection with the use of contrast media containing Iodide (51).

The absence of gall-bladder visualization in IVC is related to the age of the patient and increases from 1% (second decade) to 25% (eight decade) (52). Usually this result is caused by diseases of the gall-bladder. IVC allows the evaluation of the gall-bladder wall in the different diseases such as chole- lithiasis or chronic cholecystitis. Cholescintigraphy, however, can only demonstrate the presence or absence of gall-gladder filling. Normal subjects usually show a visualization of the gall-bladder (35) if the investigation is performed in the fasting state (35). In addition, cholescintigraphic examination is apt to give information on the "functional state" of the gall-bladder: two types of gall-bladder function can thus be differentiated that is the "bile accumulation" and the "bile excretion" type (35,53). Furthermore, even at bili- rubin levels above 4 mg% cholescintigraphic visualization of the gall-bladder is possible in parenchymal jaundice. In non-jaundiced patients Taylor et al (21) found an equal number of correct positive diagnoses with cholescintigraphy and IVC which was confirmed by the results of Kempken et al (54).

Visualization of the common bile-duct is present in about 10% (46). This percentage can be elevated to 20% if gall-bladder excretion is stimulated (46). As already mentioned, tomography of the biliary system allows visualization of the ductus choledochus in about 80% of cases (47). In contrast, cholescinti- graphy visualizes the common bile-ducts without any exception if the patient is not jaundiced (35). In parenchymal jaundice evaluation of the biliary system is still possible in 70% (55). In incomplete biliary obstruction the frequency of visualization is 65% while in complete obstructive jaundice the biliary system can no longer be evaluated (3). A comparison of IVC and cholescintigraphy re- ported by Kempken et al (54) produced the same results. A safe evaluation of the caliber of the common bile-duct is not possible by cholescintigraphy. How- ever, considering the fact that the normal width of the ductus choledochus is between 10 to 14 mm (25), it can be stated that IVC is not without any problems in the evaluation of the biliary system.

The confirmation of the presence of calculi is a domain of IVC (and sono- graphy). Some problems may be caused when the calculi are floating in the bile- ducts thus hiding in segment branches of the biliary tree. If this is the case they cannot be visualized by IVC. Cholescintigraphy is only suited to demon- strate the obstructed bile-flow caused by gall-stones. The direct proof of concretions is not possible with this procedure (21). According to Yeh et al (37) cholescintigraphy may in some cases visualize the disturbed bile-flow from segmental bile-ducts and thus give a hint of intrahepatic calculi.

To summarize these results, the following recommendations for the use of cholescintigraphy in place of IVC can be given: in contrast media intolerance and hyperthyroidism cholescintigraphy is a procedure well suited to investigate the biliary system and the gall-bladder without any side reactions. Furthermore, at bilirubin levels above 4 mg% cholescintigraphy should be used as a screening test in the differential diagnosis of jaundice. Acute cholecystitis is a further indication for cholescintigraphic procedures. In contrast, the proof of concretions and other diseases of the gall-bladder e.g. tumour and chronic inflammation require IVC.

13.6. Cholescintigraphy and endoscopic retrograde cholangio-pancreaticography (ERCP)

ERCP has become largely standardized in the last years and the success rate of probing and visualization of the biliary system is now around 62 to 85% (56,57,58,59,60). Indications for retrogarde cholangiography are bilirubin levels above 2 mg%, incomplete obstruction by calculi, benign or malignant stenosis of the papilla, obstruction of the cystic-duct, postoperative stenosis, postoperative complaints after cholecystectomy, and biliary bypass (58). The ERCP results are evaluated on hand of the diagnostic criteria of IVC. Alterations of the contour of the bile-ducts are better visualized with high density of the contrast media, concretions can safely be documented in the excretory image. Stenosis of the papilla causes diagnostic problems because of probing difficulties. Dilation of the bile-ducts alone is no safe criteria for bile obstruction. If a retention of the retrograde administered contrast media for longer than 30 minutes is observed a stenosis of the papilla may be assumed. ERCP has gained particular importance in the evaluation of complaints occuring after cholecystectomy. In 87% of the respective cases diseases of bile-ducts and/or pancreas could be demonstrated by retrograde cholangiography (58). Furthermore, in the presence of a biliary bypass ERCP allows the biliary system to be visualized.

These good results, however, are achieved with a relatively high rate of complications: according to Fölsch et al (60) in 1.6% episodes of acute pancreatitis, in 2% septic cholangitis, and in 10% abdominal complaints are observed. Some lethal complications were also reported (57).

Comparative investigations using Ida-scintigraphy and ERCP have shown that the bile-ducts were visualized in all patients without complete obstructive jaundice by cholescintigraphy and in only 69% by ERCP (17). In patients with stenosis of the papilla hepatobiliary scintigraphy was able to visualize the bile-ducts without any exception while ERCP was negative in one half of these patients. The proof of concretions however, was only possible by means of ERCP. Some cases with proven obstruction of the cystic-duct had negative iso-topic cholecystography.

As already mentioned, Miederer et al (58) have stressed the point that complaints after cholecystectomy and biliary bypass operation are the main indications for ERCP. When refering to this statement it should be mentioned that hepatobiliary scintigraphy has gained special importance in both of these diseases. Reichelt et al (61) recommends cholescintigraphy as a screening method in complaints after cholecystectomy as one half of their patients revealed scintigraphic detectable diseases of the biliary system. Furthermore, the special diagnostic indication for Ida-scintigraphy was pointed out in the case of biliary bypass operation (62) since probing of the bile-ducts is not easily performed in many cases after biliary surgery.

The following examples show a comparison of Ida and ERCP results. Fig. 11 shows the findings in a patient with stenosis of the papilla in which probing of the bile-ducts was not possible during ERCP (fig.11a) Cholescintigraphy, however, reveals the dilated common bile-duct with good excretion of the bile into the intestines which establishes that there is no significant biliary obstruction (fig.11b). Fig.12 shows the results of cholescintigraphy and ERCP in a patient with complaints some years after having undergone cholecystectomy. Both diagnostic procedures are suited to give information about the biliary system. Proof of concretions, however, is only possible with ERCP (fig.12a Ida-scintigraphy, fig.12b ERCP). Fig.13 gives an impression of the results obtained with scintigraphy (fig.13a) and ERCP fig.13b) in a patient with spontaneous fistula between the common bile-duct and the duodenum due to concretions. Detection of the fistula is only possible with ERCP, but patent bile-flow (through the fistula) is well demonstrated by cholescintigraphy.

This survey leads to the conclusion that in jaundiced patients cholescin-tigraphy should be performed prior to ERCP: if the scintigraphic diagnosis of biliary obstruction is made, PTC should be used instead of ERCP since PTC visualized the peripheric biliary system in obstruction of the common bile-duct. In biliary bypass and stenosis of the papilla cholescintigraphy can be used as a screening method and the results obtained may be used as a criterion for ERCP investigation. Cholescintigrahpy, however, is of particular importance if retrograde filling of the bile-ducts is not possible with ERCP, which is

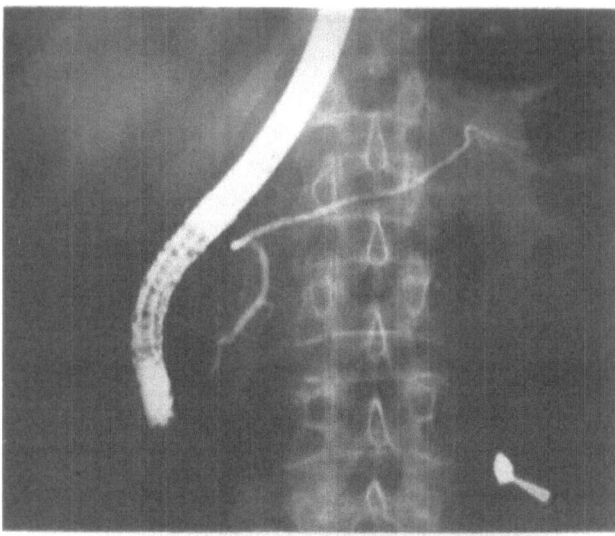

Fig. 11a

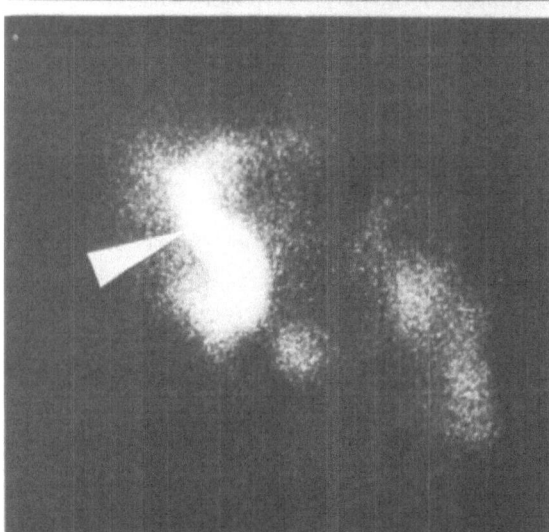

Fig. 11b

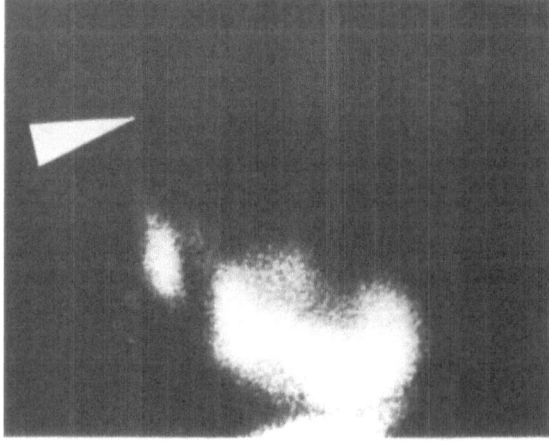

Fig.11.. Stenosis of the papilla:
a) ERCP: no probing of the common bile duct, possible.
b) Ida-scintigraphy: stenosis of the papilla, dilation of the common bile but regular discharge of the bile into the intestines.

195

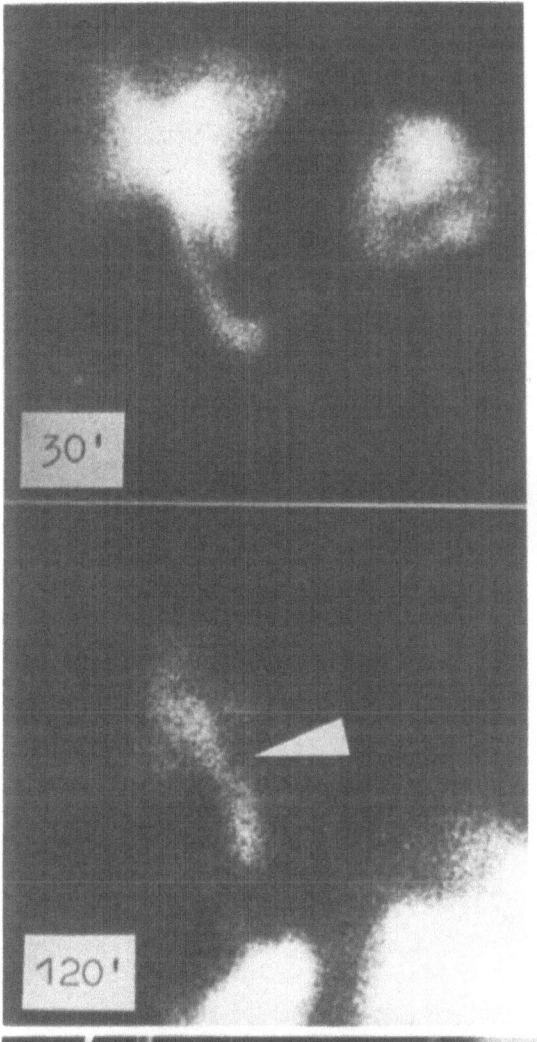

Fig. 12a

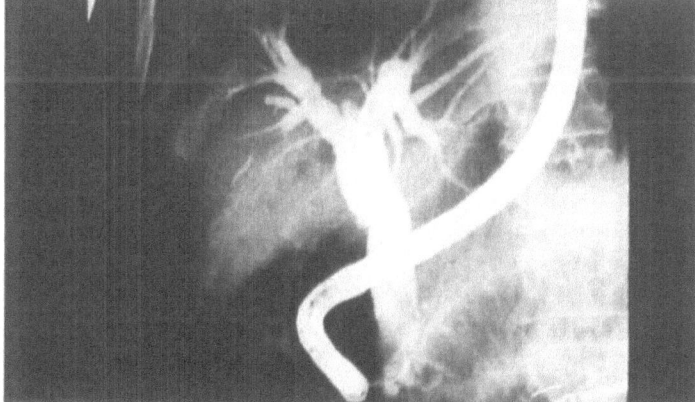

Fig. 12b

Fig.12. Complaints after cholecystectomy, prepapillary concretions:
a) Ida-scintigraphy: dilation of the bile-ducts by stenosis of the papilla, good bile discharge into GI tract.
b) ERCP: dilation of the bile-ducts, stenosis of the bile-ducts, prepapillary concretions (only visualized with ERCP).

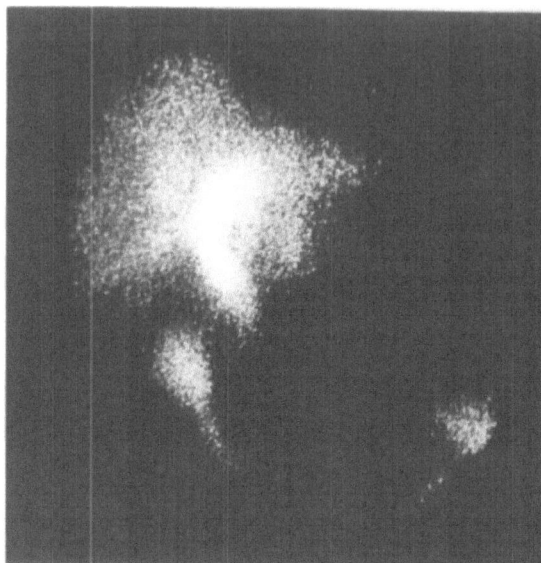

Fig. 13a

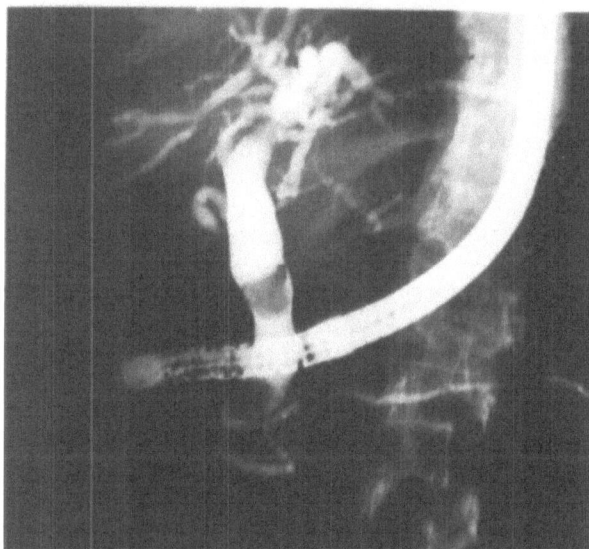

Fig. 13b

Fig.13. Spontaneous fistula between common bile-duct and duodenum because of concretions:
a) Ida-scintigraphy: dilatation of common bile-duct but good discharge of the bile.
b) ERCP: dilatation of the common bile-duct, proof of concretions and fistula.

reported to be negative in about 70% (58).

13.7.Cholescintigraphy and percutaneous transhepatic cholangiography (PTC)

PTC is the radiological method of choice in obstructive jaundice. With increasing dilatation of the biliary system puncture of the dilated bile-ducts
can successfully be performed in over 90% of cases (60,63,64,65). In parenchymal jaundice, however, the success rate drops to only 58% (63). Visualization
of non-dilated bile-ducts may be possible in about 90% if multiple punctures
are performed (66). This leads to a higher complication rate (63). In patients
with obstructive jaundice due to pre-papillary concretions or carcinoma of the
papilla PTC should be performed instead of ERCP (60). PTC offers the advantage
of demonstrating the location as well cause of the obstruction.

This highly informative, but invasive X-ray procedure is only effected
with a relative high risk: elevation of transaminases occurs in 10% of patients
and reduction of blood pressure is observed in 3% (60). Further complications
are bacteriaemia (12%) (64), cholerrhoea (3%) (63), and septic cholangitis
(0.8%) (63). According to Kreek and Balint (67), however, who collected the
results of a pilot study of more than 300 patients minor complications are
observed in 31.7% and major complications in 10.2%. The mortality rate was
0.9% and emergency surgery within 48 hours had to be performed in 3.4% (67).
Further major complications were hemorrhage (4%) and sepsis (3.1%). Absolute
contraindications for PTC are contrast media intolerance and disturbance of the
coagulation mechanism.

The previously mentioned complications should give rise to careful use of
PTC. This method should in any event only be performed if it is absolutely
necessary. Hence, bearing in mind other non-invasive methods the indications
for PTC (obstruction with dilated bile-ducts) should be carefully checked.

Cholescintigraphy together with ultrasound and CT may be used as a screening method in a combination of scintigraphic and PTC results obtained from 41
patients with obstructive jaundice gave a correct diagnosis concerning the
presence or absence of obstruction in 40 cases (17). PTC visualized the (dilated)
bile-ducts in 39 out of the 41 cases respectively. Furthermore, the site as well
as the aetiology of the obstruction could be clarified with PTC. Thus, the
absence of the bile excretion into the intestines suggested the indication for
PTC. Taylor et al (21) observed pathologic findings by cholescintigraphy in all
their patients with obstructive jaundice. They stress the point that the differential diagnosis of tumour and concretion was only possible by means of PTC. In

another report on cholescintigraphy and PTC Sty et al (68) mention the value of
Ida-derivatives in pediatric nuclear medicine. All their cases with biliary
obstruction were correctly diagnozed by this safe and non-invasive method.

By means of the following two examples the results of cholescintigraphy
and PTC are demonstrated: fig. 14 shows the results in a patient with a carcinoma
of the hepatic duct and obstructive jaundice. Cholescintigraphy shows normal
accumulation of the tracer in the liver, but compensatory renal excretion.
Delayed views up to 24 hours reveal no activity accumulation in the gastro-
intestinal tract (fig. 14a) thus leading to the diagnosis of complete obstruction.
PTC (fig. 14b) facilitated the diagnosis of the site and the aetiology (carcinoma)
of the obstruction. In fig. 15 the results in a patient with longlasting jaundice
due to carcinoma of the hepatic-duct are shown. The liver-scan with Tc^{99m}
labeled Sulphur colloid (fig.15a) reveals multiple filling defects due to
dilation of the bile-ducts. Ida-scintigraphy (fig.15b) demonstrated that there
was no accumulation of the reagent in the liver but complete compensatory renal
excretion. The combination of colloid and Ida-scintigraphy leads to the diagnosis of complete bile-duct obstruction which was confirmed by PTC (fig. 15c)

The following conclusion can be drawn from the combination of cholescintigraphy and PTC: if hepatobiliary scintigraphy leads to the diagnosis of
biliary obstruction PTC should be used instead of ERCP. However, if cholescintigraphy leads to the exclusion of obstructive jaundice there is no need to
perform PTC (and ERCP).

13.8. Cholescintigraphy and retrograde filling of the bile-ducts during gastro-intestinal X-ray after biliary bypass

Nowadays biliary bypass is performed by one or two different techniques. In
malignant obstruction choledocho-duodenostomia is used and in benign stricture
choledocho(hepatico)-jejunostomia (69). In choledocho-jejunostomia a 30 cm long
jejunal loop is interposed to avoid the reflux of ingesta. IVC and infusion
cholangiography usually yield poor results as the sphincter function of the
papilla is eliminated by the anastomosis. This results in a quick excretion of
the contrast medium with only faint visualization of the bile-ducts which allows
no clearcut diagnosis. Hence other procedures have to be used. X-ray visualization of the anastomosis after oral administration of the contrast medium is
difficult because of the jejunum interponate. The reflux of contrast media
during gastrointestinal X-ray is caused by abdominal pressure. Later the
discharge of the contrast media can be utilized to evaluate the function of the
biliary bypass.

The difficulties mentioned here gave rise to the inclusion of cholescintigraphy in the evaluation of the bile-ducts and the anastomosis after biliary
bypass (62,70). Retrograde filling of the bile-ducts after orally administered
contrast media resulted in visualization of the bile-ducts in only 80% of the
cases while cholescintigraphy was successful in all patients (62). In most of
the patients with no retrograde filling hepatobiliary scintigraphy revealed
dilated bile-ducts which was interpreted as a moderate biliary obstruction (62).
In these cases diagnosis was only possible with cholescintigraphy. This method
is therefore highly useful to evaluate the function of a biliary bypass as the
scintigraphic proof of bile discharge is a proof of the good function of the
anastomosis.

By means of two examples the value of cholescintigraphy in biliary bypass
can be illustrated: fig.16 shows a moderate dilation of the bile-ducts in a
biliary bypass (fig.16a: cholescintigraphy, fig.16b: retrograde filling with
contrast media). Fig.17 shows the findings in a patient with markedly dilated
bile-ducts but a good discharge of bile (fig.17a) hepatobiliary scintigraphy,
fig.17b: X-ray, retrogade filling).

These results lead to the conclusion that cholescintigraphy is of particular value in patients with biliary bypass when retrograde filling with contrast
media during gastrointestinal X-ray is not possible (62,70).

13.9.Cholescintigraphy and angiography

Indications for liver angiography are described in detail in the book of
McNulty (71). There are three diseases of the liver in which combination of
angiography and cholescintigraphy may be helpful; these are space-occupying
lesions, liver trauma, and jaundice.

Cholescintigraphy of focal lesions is reported on in detail elsewhere in
this book: the combination of Ida-scintigraphy and angiography facilitates the
differential diagnosis in some rare cases of liver tumours, e.g. hepatic adenoma
and focal nodular hyperplasia of the liver.

Angiographic investigation of the biliary tract is one method of demonstrating the gall-bladder when there is cystic-duct obstruction (71). Normally the
entire gall-bladder wall is opacified in the hepatogram phase of the angiogram.
In some tumours of the gall-bladder a pathological circulation is present (71).
Angiography can thus verify the causes of negative isotopic cholecystography.
Indications for selective liver angiography (as may be established by cholescintigraphy) are nodular hepatomegaly, known primary tumour site, suspected

pancreatic carcinoma, recent abdominal trauma, jaundice, and bleeding (71).

The presence of perihepatic, subcapsular, or intrahepatic aneurysms or arteriovenous fistulae after penetrating or non-penetrating liver trauma may be demonstrated by angiography (71). Cholescintigraphy, however, may permit the visualization of biliary fistulae trauma (72). It would appear therefore that there are only some rare cases in which hepatobiliary scintigraphy can help to clarify angiographic findings or in which angiography should be used in the further diagnostics of cholescintigraphic findings.

13.10.Cholescintigraphy and laboratory tests

Liver tissue contains a lot of enzymes of which some are only to be found in this organ, so called liver specific enzymes. Three groups of liver enzymes can be differentiated (73):

a. Secretory enzymes are synthetized in the hepatocytes and secreted into the plasma. Some of these are cholinesterases and coagulation factors. The decrease of these enzymes in the plasma leads to the diagnosis of severe parenchymal damage.

b. Excretory enzymes such as alkaline phosphateses are excreted with the bile. Their elevated plasma levels may be indicative of biliary obstruction.

c. Indicator enzymes are present in the cytoplasma of the hepatocytes. Their penetration through the membrane into plasma is indicative of acute parenchymal damage. The most important indicator enzymes are glutamata-pyruvate transaminasis (GPT), glutamate-oxalacetate transaminasis (GOT), and lactate dehydrogenasis (LDH).

Further important parameters are gamma-glutamyl transferasis (gamma-GT), bilirubin, ESR and leucocytes. In addition to these parameters special quotients (De-Ritis) from the transaminases, e.g. GOT/GPT or gamma GT/GOT can be derived, which are of high value in the differential diagnosis of jsundice. The laboratory findings in the different diseases of liver and biliary tract are as follows:

Acute cholecystitis is a clinical diagnosis. Laboratory tests are not indicative but can be of some value (slightly elevated levels of bilirubin, transaminases, ESR, and leucocytes). Acute cholecystitis is characterized by negative isotopic cholecystography..

Obstructive jaundice reveals a typical enzyme pattern within one week of the onset of the disease: transaminases are increased up to the 10 fold of their normal values (25), the De-Ritis-quotient is low (25). At the end of the

first week of the disease the transaminase levels are decreasing to normal
values and an elevation of the cholestasis-specific enzymes (gamma GT, alkaline
phosphatases) as well as of bilirubin is observed. This is the time at which
"cholescintigraphy is a sensitive and reliable method for detecting the
functional abnormality of obstruction, before the morphologic change of
dilatation is seen in ultrasonography and even before the liver function test
are abnormal" (24). The prothrombin level is only decreasing after several days
when resorption of vitamine K is no longer present. If biliary obstruction is
caused by cholangitis the parameters of inflammation are observed in addition.
These are leucocytosis, elevated ESR, and elevation of alpha-2-globulines. The
findings of cholescintigraphy in obstructive jaundice have been described in
detail elsewhere. From animal experiments Bähre et al (74) were able to re-
produce the laboratory and cholescintigraphic findings in obstructive jaundice.

Parenchymal jaundice is characterized by the intense increase of the
transaminase to more than 1000 IE whilst bilirubin and alkaline phosphatase
show only moderately elevated levels. The alteration of the De-Ritis-quotient is
related to the aetiology of parenchymal damage (25). The results of Bähre et al
(74) showed similar results in galactosamine-induced hepatitis: bilirubin was
elevated to 20 to 30 fold levels, GPT, however, to 300 fold levels. In spite of
these values accumulation of Ida in the hepatocytes as well as biliary
excretion could be observed so that diagnosis of parenchymal jaundice was
possible in all animals. A close correlation of bilirubin levels with the
urinary excretion of Ida was reported by Huemer et al (75).

In summary it can be stated that parenchymal and obstructive jaundice are
characterized by specific enzyme patterns. In many cases, however, diagnosis is
not possible on the basis of laboratory tests alone. In these cases cholescintigraphy may help to establish the correct diagnosis which is possible in more
than 90% of all cases (3,18).

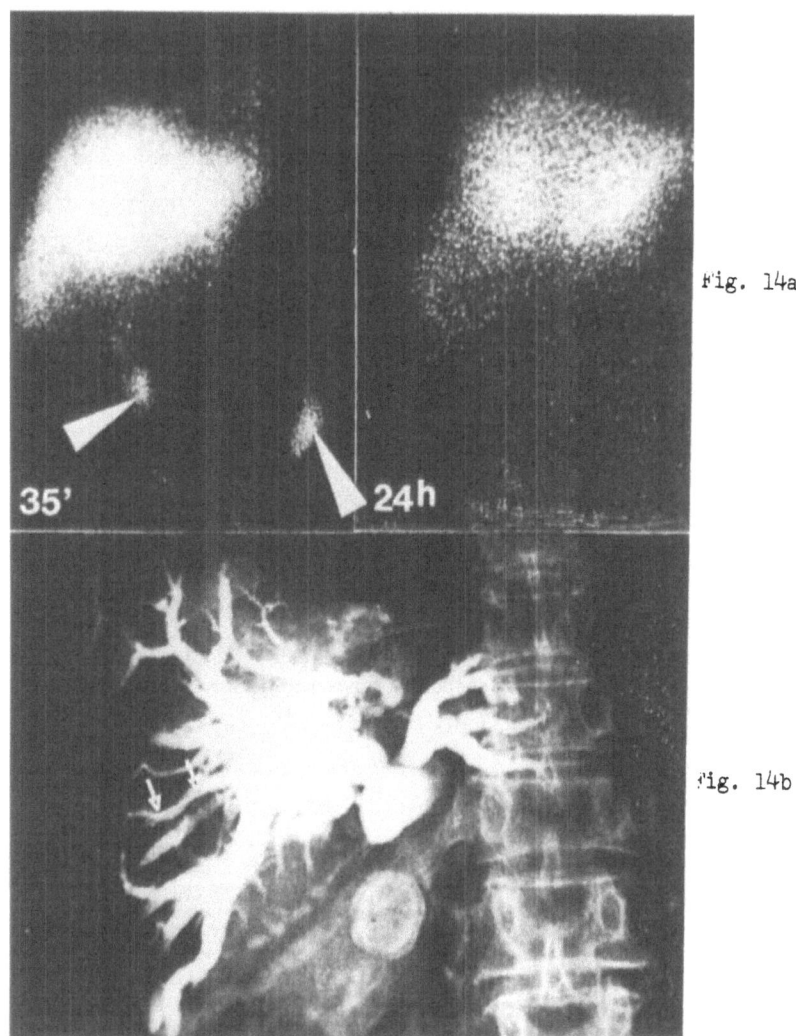

Fig. 14a

Fig. 14b

Fig.14. Carcinoma of the hepatic-duct:
a) Ida-scintigraphy: regular tracer accumulation in the liver as well as
compensatory renal excretion; no bile discharge into the GI tract up to 24
hours post injection.
b) PTC: dilated bile-ducts because of malignant stenosis of the hepatic-duct.

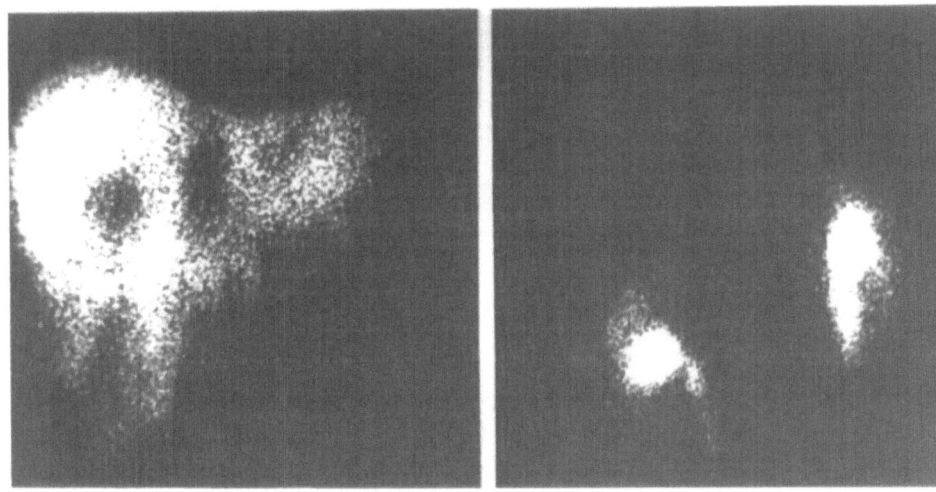

Fig. 15a

Fig. 15b

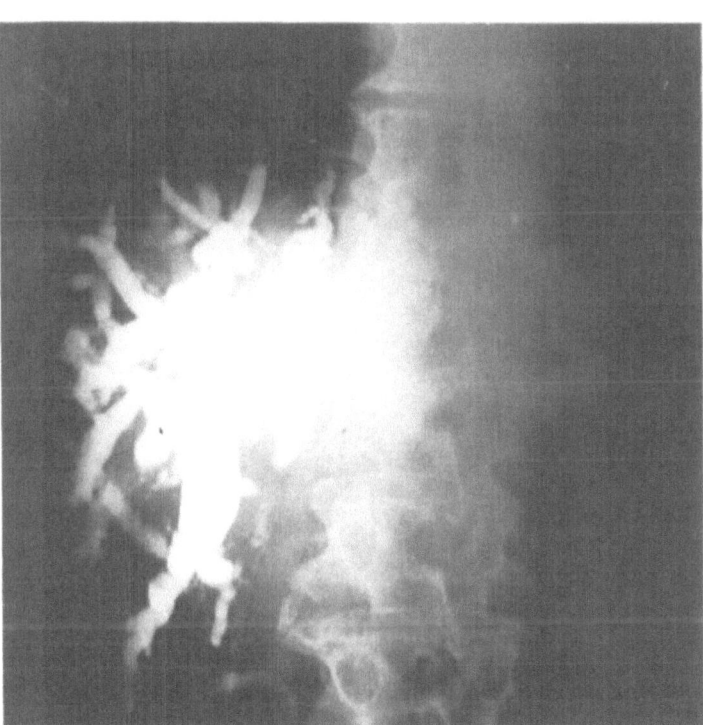

Fig. 15c

Fig.15. Longlasting jaundice because of carcinoma of the hepatic duct:
a) Liver-scan with Sulphur colloid: multiple filling defects due to dilated
bile-ducts.
b) Ida-scintigraphy: complete renal excretion of the tracer, no accumulation
in the liver.
c) PTC: malignant stenosis of the hepatic-duct with dilation of bile-ducts.

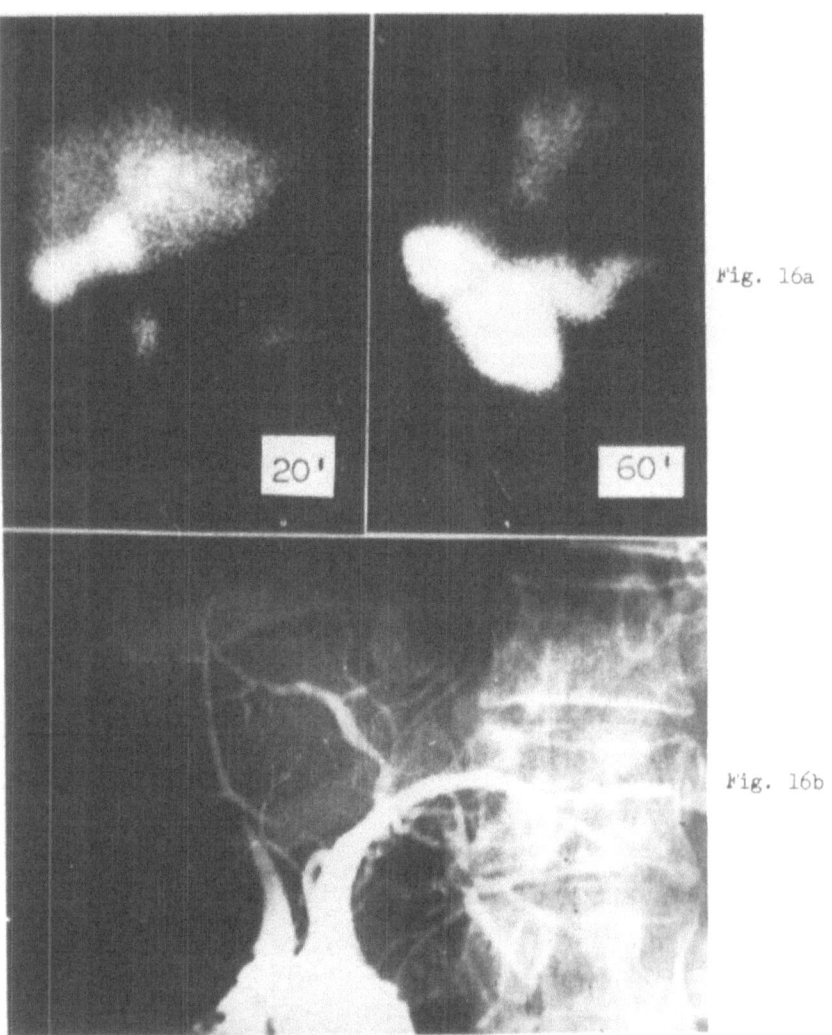

Fig. 16a

Fig. 16b

Fig.16. Biliary bypass:
Slightly dilated bile-ducts with retention of the tracer but regular bile
discharge (a: Ida-scintigraphy, b: gastrointestinal X-ray).

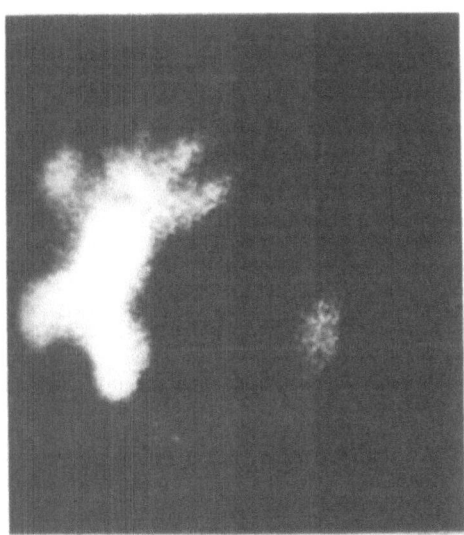

Fig. 17a

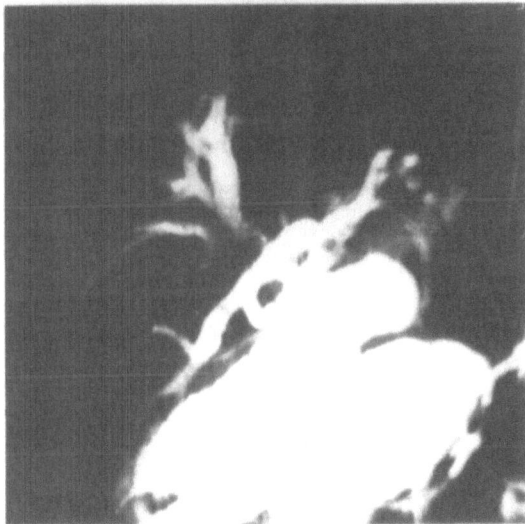

Fig. 17b

Fig. 17 Biliary bypass:
Markedly dilated bile-ducts with clearly visible retention of the tracer but
good bile discharge (a: Ida-Scintigraphy, b: gastrointestinal X-ray).

REFERENCES

1. Matolo N, Stadalnik M, Krohn RC, Biliary tract scanning with Tc-99m-pyri-
   doxylideneglutamate: A new gall-bladder scanning agent. Surgery 80:317, 1976.

2. Biersack HJ, Thelen M, Breuel HP, ^{99m}Tc-Hepatobida zur Funktionsszintigraphie der Leber - Simultanvergleich mit ^{131}I-Bromsulphan durch Dopper-
   tracer-Sequenz-szintigraphie. NucComp. 8:6, 1977.

3. Biersack HJ, Thelen M, Lindstaedt H, Hepatobiliäre Funktionsszintigraphie
   mit ^{99m}Tc-markierten Ida-Derivaten bei Leber- und Gallenwegserkrankungen.
   Inn. Med. 6:56, 1979.

4. Middendorp UG, Klinische Aspekte des Verschluss-Ikterus, Bern, Stuttgart,
   Wien, Huber, 1979.

5. Biersack HJ, Thelen M, Knopp R, Funktionsszintigraphie der Leber und der
   Gallenwege mit ^{99m}Tc-Diäthyl-Ida. Röfo 27:422, 1977.

6. Wilcox JR, Green JP, Moniot AL, Functional evaluation of a hepatic scintigraphic defect using ultrasound and a fatty meal: case report. J. nucl. Med.
   18:32, 1977.

7. Hünermann B, Albert JP, Winkler C, Prinzipien der szintigraphischen Leber-
   diagnostiek. Med. Klin. 67:1288, 1972.

8. McAfee JG, Ause RG, Wagner HN, Diagnostic value of scintillation scanning
   of the liver. Arch. intern. Med. 116:95, 1965.

9. Biersack HJ, Helpap B, Bell E, Zur Treffsicherheit der Leberszintigraphie
   bei focalen Lebererkrankungen - ein Vergleich mit dem Obduktionsbefund
   anhand von 159 Fällen. Nucl. Med. 18:177, 1979.

10. Dewburry KC, Clark B, The accuracy of ultrasound in the detection of
    cirrhosis of the liver. Brit. J. Radiol. 52:945, 1979.

11. Heilmann S, Sonografie, Laparoskopie und Histologie bei diffusen Lederer-
    krankungen. Münch. med. Wschr. 122:339, 1980.

12. Albertson KW, Leopold IR, Liver. In: Abdominal gray scale ultrasonography.
    Goldberg BB (ed), New York, London, Sydney, Toronto, Wiley & Sons J, 1977,
    p. 103.

13. Rettenmeier G, Seitz KH, Ultraschalluntersuchung bei Ikterus. Dtsch. med.
    Wschr. 102:1559, 1977.

14. Schneekloth G, Jäger M, Bedeutung der Sonographie bei der Abklärung einer
    unklaren Cholestase. Schweiz. med. Wschr. 109:517, 1979.

15. Sabel JS, Graham DY, Davis RE, The value of gray scale ultrasound in the
    differential diagnosis of surgical and nonsurgical jaundice. Amer. J.
    Gastroent. 69:149, 1978.

16. Dewburry KC, Joseph AEA, Hayes S, Ultrasound in the evaluation and diagnosis
    of jaundice. Brit. J. Radiol. 52:276, 1979.

17. Biersack HJ, Lindstaedt H, Thelen M, Hepatobiliäre Funktionsszintigraphie
    (HBFS) mit Ida-Derivaten - ihre Bedeutung im Vergleich zu endoskopisch-
    retrograder Cholangiographie (ERC) und perkutan-transhepatischer Cholangio-
    graphie (PTC). In: Radioaktive Isotope in Klinik und Forschung. Höfer RH,
    Bergmann J, (eds), Wien, Egermann, 1980, p. 99.

18. Pauwels S, Perit L, Schoutens A, Clinical role of ^{99m}Tc-diethyl-Ida scintigraphy in jaundiced patients. J. nucl. Med. 20:685, 1979.

19. Ryan J, Isikoff M, Nagle C, The combined use of ^{99m}Tc-Hida and ultrasound in differential diagnosis of jaundice. J. nucl. Med. 17:545, 1976.

20. Klingensmith WC, Johnson M, Kuni CC, Complimentary role of Tc-99m-diethyl-Ida und ultrasound in large and small duct biliary tract obstruction. J. nucl. Med. 21:41, 1980.

21. Taylor TV, Sumerling MD, Carter DC, An evaluation of ^{99m}Tc-labelled Hida in hepatobiliary scanning. Brit. J. Surg. 67:325, 1980.

22. Suarez CA, Block F, Bernstein D, The role of Hida-Pipida scanning in diagnosing cystic duct obstruction. Ann. Surg. 191:391, 1980.

23. Prokop EK, Technetium-99m Pipida and Technetium-99m-sulfur colloid liver scanning combined with ultrasound in the evaluation of patients with jaundice. J. nucl. Med. 20:600, 1979.

24. Weissmann HS, Rosenblatt RR, Sugarman LA, Early diagnosis of acute common bile duct obstruction by Tc-99m-Ida (iminodiacetic acid) cholescintigraphy. J. nucl. Med. 21:41, 1980.

25. Malchow H, Frommhold W, Jenss H, Diagnostik bei Erkrankungen der Gallenwege. Internist 21:565, 1980.

26. Anderson JC, Harned RK, Gray scale ultrasonography of the gallbladder: an evaluation of accuracy and report of additional ultrasound signs. Amer. J. Roentgenol. 129:957, 1977.

27. Arnon S, Rosenqvist CJ, Gray scale cholecystosonography: an evaluation of accuracy. Amer. J. Roentgenol. 127:817, 1976.

28. Crade M, Taylor KJW, Rosenfield AT, Surgical and pathological correlation of cholecystosonography and cholecystography. Amer. J. Roentgenol. 131:227, 1978.

29. Lawson TL, Gray scale cholecystosonography. Radiology 122:247, 1977.

30. Cooperberg PL, Burhenne HJ, Real time ultrasonography. Diagnostic technique of choice in calculous gallbladder disease. New. Engl. J. Med. 302:1277, 1980.

31. Paré EA, Shaffer EA, Rosenthall L, Non-visualization of the gallbladder by ^{99m}Tc-Hida cholescintigraphy as evidence of cholecystitis. Canad. Med. Ass. J. 118:384, 1978.

32. Weissmann HS, Frank M, Rosenblatt R, Correlation of Tc-99m-Hida with anatomic imaging in patients with hepatobiliary disease. J. nucl. Med. 19:738, 1978.

33. Freeman LM, Comments. In: Radioaktive Isotope in Klinik und Forschung. Vol. 14. Part. 2. Höfer RH, Bergmann J (eds), Wien, Egermann, 1980, p. 566.

34. Tjen HSLM, Die Choleszintigraphie und die Gallenblase. In: Hepatobiliäre Funktionsszintigraphie mit Ida-Derivaten. Biersack HJ, Mahlstedt J (eds), Darmstadt, G-I-T/E Giebler, 1978, p. 125.

35. Biersack HJ, Breuel HP, Thelen M, Beurteilungskriterien der hepatobiliären Funktionsszintigraphie mit ^{99m}Tc-markiertem Diäthyl-Ida- Befunde bei Lebergesunden. Röfo 130:689, 1979.

36. Braun B, Schwerk W, Ultraschalldiagnostiek der Cholelithiasis. Ein Vergleich mit röntgenologischen Untersuchungsverfahren. Dtsch. med. Wschr. 103:1101, 1978.

37. Yeh SH, Liu OK, Huang MJ, Technetium-99m-Pyridoxylideneglutamate (Tc-99m-PG) sequential scintiphotography in the detection of intrahepatic stones. J. nucl. Med. 18:635, 1977.

38. Stadler HW, Rödl W, Fuchs HF, Was bringt die Computertomographie bei Erkrankungen des Verdauungstrakts? Dtsch. Ärztebl. 77:319, 1980.

39. Scherer U, Lissner J, Brall N, Computertomographie der Leber - Treffsicherheit der Methode bei bioptischer gesicherten Diagnosen. Röfo 130:531, 1979.

40. Levitt R, Sagel SS, Stanley RJ, Accuracy of computed tomography of the liver anf biliary tract. Radiology 124:123, 1977.

41. Frühling J, Osteaux M, Correlation between liverscintigraphy and computed tomography in the detection of liver metastases. Eur. J. Nucl. Med. 3:169, 1978.

42. Grossman ZD, Wistow BW, Bryan PJ, Radionuclide imaging, computed tomography, and gray scale ultrasonography of the liver: a comparative study. J. nucl. Med. 18:327, 1977.

43. Scherer U, Büll U, Rothe R, Computerized tomography and nuclear imaging of the liver. A comparative study in 83 cases. Eur. J. Nucl. Med. 3:71, 1978.

44. MacCarty RL, Wahner HW, Stephens DH, Retrospective comparison of radionuclide scans and tomography of the liver and pancreas. Amer. J. Roentgenol. 129:23, 1977.

45. Bryan PJ, Dinn WM, Grossman ZD, Correlation of computed tomography, gray scale ultrasonography, and radionuclide imaging of the liver in detecting space-occupying processes. Radiology 124:387, 1977.

46. Hippéli R, Eibach E, Rationelle kombinierte Röntgenuntersuchung von Gallenblase und Magen. Leber, Magen, Darm 9:111, 1979.

47. Grauthoff H, Thelen M, Peters M, Vergleich der Wertigkeit von intravenösem bzw. Infusionscholangiogramm sowie intraoperativem und Tomocholangiogramm. Röfo 127:575, 1977.

48. Stauch GW, Löhr E, Paar G, Das "konventionelle" Infusionscholangiozystogramm. Med. Welt. 26:106, 1975.

49. Ordnung W, Müting D, Gallenkontrastmittel bei chronischen Leberkrankheiten. Med. Klin. 74:149, 1979.

50. Winckler K, Lebernekrosen nach Infusions-Cholangiographie. Dtsch. med. Wschr. 103:420, 1978.

51. Breuel HP, Breuel C, Emrich D, Veränderungen der Schilddrüsenfunktion durch Röntgenkontrastmittel bei Schilddrüsengesunden. Med. Klin. 74:1492, 1979.

52. Strik WO, Züchner F, Fleischner K, Ergebnisse von 11 699 Cholezysto- und Cholangiographien. Therapiewoche 26:7462, 1976.

53. Reichelt HG, Nuklearmedizinische Leber- und Gallenwegsdiagnostik mit dem hepatotropen cholophilen Radiopharmakon ^{99m}Tc-Diäthyl-Ida (EHIDA). NucComp. 9:86, 1978.

54. Kempken H, Langhammer H, Rupp N, Die hepatobiliäre Funktionsszintigraphie mit 99mTc-Diäthyl-Hida im Vergleich zur Röntgendiagnostik. In: Nuklearmedizin. Klinische Bedeutung der nuklearmedizinischen Diagnostik und Therapie. Schmidt HAE, Ortiz Berrocal J, (eds), Stuttgart, New York, Schattauer, 1979, p. 588.

55. Biersack HJ, Bruel HP, Altland H, Morphologische und funktionelle Beurteilungskriterien der hepatobiliären Funktionsszintigraphie mit 99mTc-Diäthyl-Ida bei Parenchymikterus. Nucl. Med. 18:204, 1979.

56. Belolahvek D, Koch H, Rösch W, Five years experience in endoscopic retrograde cholangiopancreatography. Endoscopy 8:115, 1976.

57. Miederer SE, Stadelmann O, Löffler A, Die endoskopische retrograde Cholangio-Pankreatikographie (ERCP): Indikation, Technik, Wertigkeit und Risiko. Lcbcr, Magen, Darm 4:187, 1974.

58. Miederer SE, Mayershofer R, Fricke G, Der diagnostische Wert der endoskopischen retrograden Cholangiographie. Therapiewoche 30:7911, 1980.

59. Sauerbruch T, Wotzka R, Rummel T, Diagnostischer Wert von Sonographie und ERCP. Münch. med. Wschr. 121:1539, 1979.

60. Fölsch UR, Wurbs D, Classen M, Vergleich der perkutanen transhepatischen Cholangiographie und der endoskopischen retrograden Cholangiopankreatographie. Dtsch. med. Wschr. 104:625, 1979.

61. Reichelt HG, Stender HS, Schmidt FW, Hepatobiliäre Sequenzszintigraphie - Fortschritte in der Abklärung von Rest- und Nachbeschwerden Cholezystektomierter. Röfo 128:451, 1978.

62. Biersack HJ, Siedek M, Franken T, Funktionsprüfung biliodigestiver Anastomosen mit 99mTc-markierten Ida-Derivaten. In: Hepatobiliäre Funktionsszintigraphie mit Ida-Derivaten. Biersack HJ, Mahlstedt J, (eds), Darmstadt, G-I-T/E, Giebler, 1978, p. 169.

63. Dammermann R, Zilly W, Trülzsch D, Die Bedeutung der perkutanen transhepatischen Cholangiographie (PTC) mit ultradünner Nadel in der Differentialdiagnose der Cholestase. Dsch. med. Wschr. 103:371, 1978.

64. Ferucci JT, Wittenberg J, Refinements in Chiba needle transhepatic cholangiography. Amer. J. Roentgenol. 129:11, 1977.

65. Gold RP, Casarella WJ, Stern G, Transhepatic cholangiography: the radiological method of choice in suspected obstructive jaundice. Radiology 133:39, 1979.

66. Okuda K, Tanikawa K, Imura T, Non-surgical, percutaneous transhepatic cholangiography. Diagnostic significance in medical problems of the liver. Amer. J. dig. Dis. 19:21, 1974.

67. Kreek MJ, Balint JA, "Skinny needle" cholangiography - results of a pilot study of a voluntary prospective method for gathering risk data on new procedures. Gatroenterology 78:598, 1980.

68. Sty JR, Babbitt DP, Robert A, 99mTc-Pipida biliary imaging in children. Clin. Nucl. Med. 4:315, 1979.

69. Zenker R, Berchtold R, Hamelmann H, Allgemeine und spezielle chirurgische Operationslehre. Vol. VII/1. Berlin, Heidelberg, New York, Springer, 1975.

70. Reichelt HG, Pichlmayr L, Nuklearmedizinisch- diagnostische Exploration biliodigestiver Anastomosen. Röfo 127:567, 1977.

71. McNulthy JG, Radiology of the liver Saunders Company WB, Philadelphia, London, Toronto, 1977.

72. Biersack HJ, Mahlstedt J, Hepatobiliäre Funktionsszintigraphie mit Ida-Derivaten. Darmstadt, G-I-T/E, Giebler, 1978.

73. Schmid M, Leber. In: Klinische Pathophysiologie. Siegenthaler (ed), Stuttgart, Thieme, 1970, p. 677.

74. Bähre M, Biersack HJ, Hofmann S, Cholescintigraphy in experimentally induced obstructive and parenchymatous jaundice. In: Progress in Radiopharmacology. Vol. 1. Cox PH (ed), Amsterdam, Elsevier/North-Holland Biomedical Press, 1979, p. 195.

75. Hümer T, Falkensammer M, Judmaier G, Leberfunktionsszintigraphie mit ^{99m}Tc-Hida: klinische Bedeutung im Vergleich zu chemisch-radiologischen Untersuchungsmethoden. In: Nuklearmedizin - Klinische Bedeutung nuklearmedizinischer Diagnostik und Therapie. Schmidt HAE, Ortiz Berrocal J (eds), Stuttgart, New York, Schattauer, 1979, p. 602.

14. ORTHOTOPIC TRANSPLANTATION OF LIVER AND BILE DRAINAGE

H.G. REICHELT

Despite growing experimental and clinical experience on liver transplantation with regard to immunological problems there are still surgical technical
obstacles including the reconstruction of the bile pathways. Following transplantation as well as during a rejection there is a change in bile production
including a change in the composition of bile acids. In the case of impaired
bile drainage bile acids may fall out and cause cholestasis. Immuno-suppression
therapy with its risk of infectious diseases then may lead to cholangitis.
Immunosuppression therapy may itself (Azathioprin[R]) lead to cholestasis by increasing bile viscosity. In liver transplant surgery therefore its imperative
to apply a free bile drainage. Different techniques of biliobiliary and biliodigestive anastomoses are applicable:
- cholecystoduodenostomy
- choledocho- cholecystojejunostomy (figs. 1a - d)
- end-to-end anastomosis with interposition of the gallbladder (Calne) (figs.
  2a - c)
    Cholescintigraphy can differentiate between hepatocellular jaundice (e.g.
immunosuppression)and obstruction. Impairment of bile drainage - stasis,
obstruction, dysfunction and the anastomized loop all causes of cholangitis can
be detected and fairly well localized.

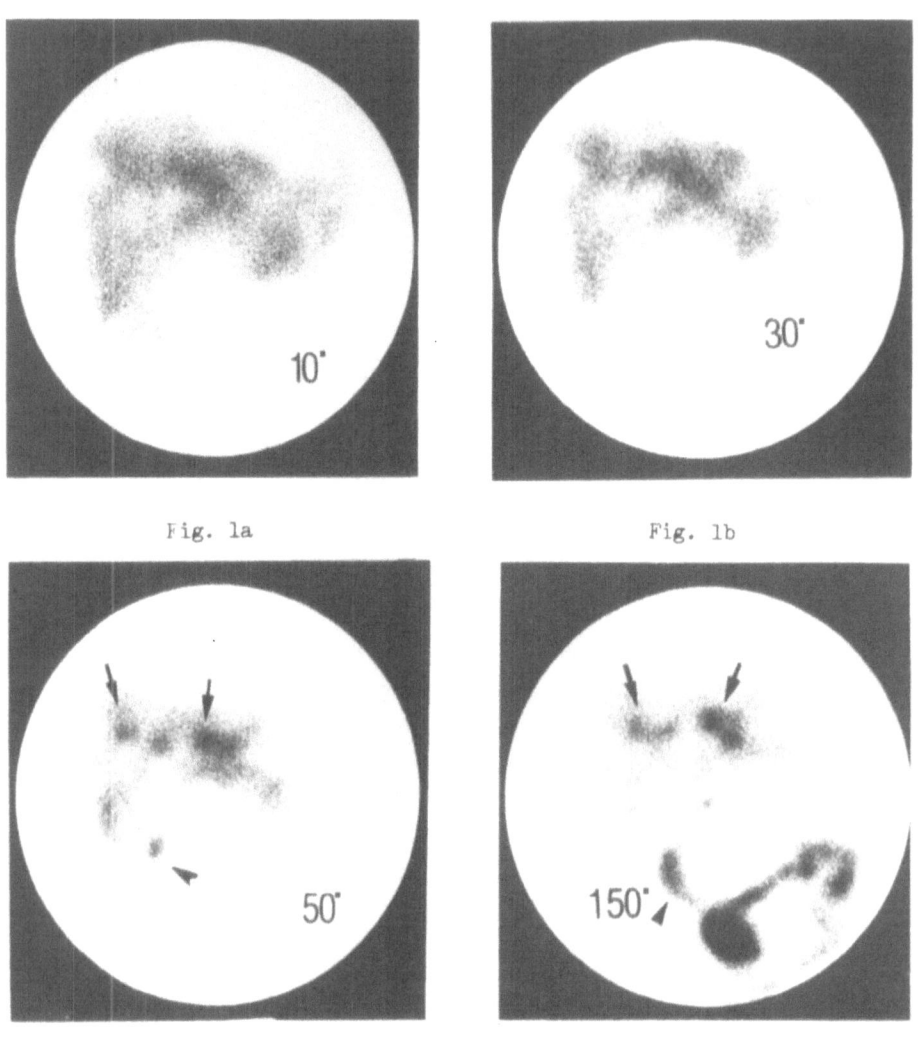

Fig. 1a   Fig. 1b

Fig. 1c   Fig. 1d

Fig. 1a-d. Cholescintigram (10, 30, 50 and 150 min): metastases cause multiple large parenchymal defects; stasis of activity in intrahepatic bile ducts following slight obstruction by the metastases; free bile drainage via cholecysto-jejunostomy (◄─intrahepatic bile ducts, ◄ gallbladder, ◄ bowel).

Fig. 1c. Livertransplant (same patient as fig. 4) - 4 month. after transplantation multiple large metastases of the hepatocellular carcinoma - cholecysto-jejunostomy; bilirubin 3 mg/100 ml.

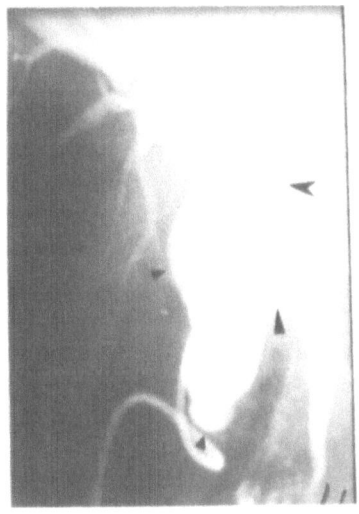

Fig. 2a

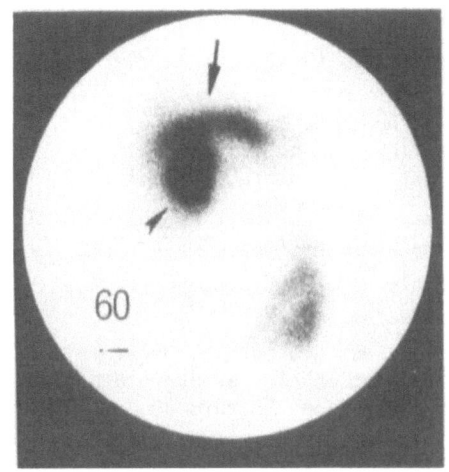

Fig. 2b

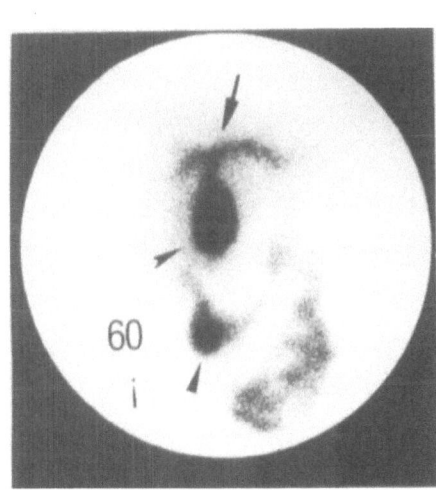

Fig. 2c

Fig. 10a. Cholangiogram via transanastomotic drain: anatomical situation; anastomoses of choledochi with the gallbladder (◀ and ◀).

Fig. 10b. End-to-end anastomosis with interposition of the gallbladder (Calne) in liver transplant.

Fig. 10b, c. Cholescintigram in supine (·—) and up-right (!) position (60 min): stasis and reflux of activity in supine position (◀—intrahepatic bile ducts; ◀ gallbladder); improved bile drainage in up-right position (◀ bowel).

LITERATURE

1. Dewanjee MK, Fliegel D, Treves S, Davis MA, 99mTc-labeled tetracycline: a new radiopharmaceutical for renal imaging. J. nucl. Med. 13:427, 1972.

2. Iga T, Awazn S, Hanano M, Nogami H, Pharmacokinetic studies of biliary excretion. I. Comparison of the excretion behaviour of pharmacokinetic studies. Chem. pharm. Bull. 19:273, 1971.

3. Reichelt HG, Pichlmayr R, Nuklearmedizinische-diagnostische Exploration biliodigestiver Anastomosen. Röfo 127, 6:567, 1977.

4. Reichelt HG, Funktionsgestörte Roux-Y-Schlinge bei biliodigestiven Anastomosen. Chirurg 48, p. 777, 1977.

5. Reichelt HG, Bockhorn H, Hepato-biliäre Sequenz-Szintigraphie. Eine diagnostische Möglichkeit zur Überprüfung des Galleabflusses nach orthotoper Lebertransplantation. Chirurg 49, p. 491, 1978.

6. Smith R, Sherlock S, Surgery of the gallbladder and bile ducts, London, Butterworths, 1964.

7. Starzl TE, Marchio TL, Kaulla K,v, Herrmann G, Brittain RS, Waddel WR, Homotransplantation of the liver in humans. Surg. Gynec. Obstet. 117:659, 1963.

CONCLUSION

P.H. COX

Cholescintigraphy is a sensitive non invasive technique which can be used
to evaluate a wide spectrum of hepatobiliary diseases. Its use is not limited
by bilirubin levels and there are no known contraindications. Of the reagents
available Tc^{99m} Diethyl-Ida appears to be the reagent of choice although other
Ida-derivatives with similar short liver transit times may also be effective.

PROTOCOL

A recommended basic protocol for cholescintigraphy is given below:

- Reagent: Tc^{99m} Diethyl-Ida
- Dose: 185 MBq (5 mCi)
- Premedication: none patient should fast for 4 hours prior to the study
- Procedure: with the patient lying prone on his back the head of the
gamma camera is positioned to include the liver and upper abdomen (for intestin-
al and kidney activity) in the field plus myocardium

The Technetium-Diethyl-Ida is injected intravenously and serial scintigrams
are made for 45 minutes. At the same time computer records are made (90 records
of 30 seconds) for the generation of time activity curves and eventually
functional images.

If at the end of the study there is no intestinal activity visible follow-
up scintigrams should be made 24 hours post injection.

In the presence of intestinal activity gastric reflux can be controlled by
placing the patient on his left side for 5 minutes and then preparing an antero-
posterior scintigram. The gall-bladder emptying can be observed by giving the
patient a fatty meal or oral stimulant, at the end of the study.

Radiation dose (mGy)

- liver   4.5
- gall-bladder   55

- intestines:
  large: 17.5
  small: 9.5
- kidneys: 3.0
- ovaries: 3.5
- total body: 1.0

SUBJECT INDEX